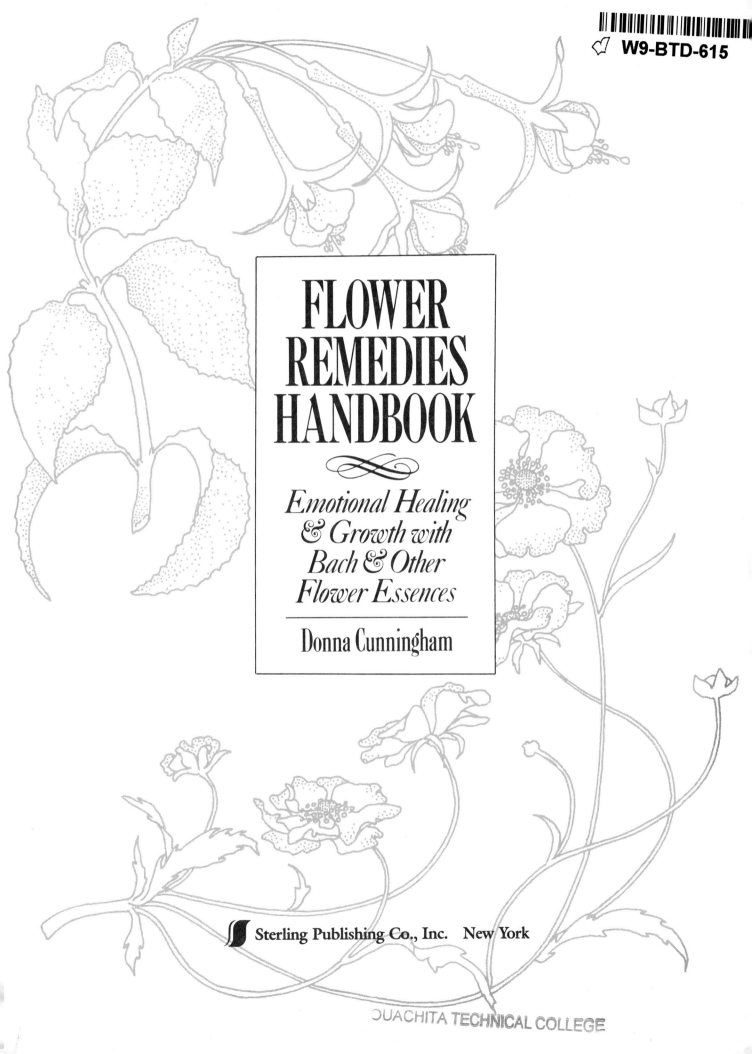

W9-BTD-615

FLOWER REMEDIES HANDBOOK

*Emotional Healing
& Growth with
Bach & Other
Flower Essences*

Donna Cunningham

Sterling Publishing Co., Inc.   New York

OUACHITA TECHNICAL COLLEGE

This book is dedicated to Dr. John Fogarty, to Charles Whitefeather, and to my half-Comanche grandfather, Arthur Hedges, who was exceptionally gifted with plants.

Library of Congress Cataloging-in-Publication Data

Cunningham, Donna, 1942–
    Flower remedies handbook: emotional healing & growth with Bach
and other flower essences / Donna Cunningham.
        p.   cm.
    Includes bibliographical references and index.
    ISBN 0-8069-8204-7
    1. Flowers—Therapeutic use—Handbooks, manuals, etc.   I. Title.
RX615.F55C86   1991
615′.321—dc20
                                                                        91-16851
                                                                        CIP

10 9 8 7 6 5 4 3

© 1992 by Donna Cunningham
Published by Sterling Publishing Company, Inc.
387 Park Avenue South, New York, N.Y. 10016
Distributed in Canada by Sterling Publishing
% Canadian Manda Group, P.O. Box 920, Station U
Toronto, Ontario, Canada M8Z 5P9
Distributed in Great Britain and Europe by Cassell PLC
Villiers House, 41/47 Strand, London WC2N 5JE, England
Distributed in Australia by Capricorn Link Ltd.
P.O. Box 665, Lane Cove, NSW 2066
Manufactured in the United States of America
All rights reserved

Sterling ISBN 0-8069-8204-7 Trade

Acknowledgments

To Matthew Wood, Patricia Kaminski, and Richard Katz, for permission to quote from their writings.

To the various flower remedy companies and those responsible for making the essences and researching their meanings, for permission to quote from their findings.

To my editor, Sheila Anne Barry, for suggesting this book and making it a reality.

To Sherry Mestel, for being there in the beginning and generously teaching me about the remedies.

To the flower angels, for their patient desire to teach and heal their human relatives.

To Scarecrow Press, for permission to reprint the flower calendar from Gertrude Jobes's *Dictionary of Mythology, Folklore, and Symbols*.

To Carol Lipton, for the use of her original drawings of sagebrush, comfrey, star of Bethlehem, and centaury.

To Joan Columbus, for her original drawings of agrimony, holly, rhubarb, Sturt desert pea, and willow.

The following illustrations used in this book are from the Dover Publications copyright-free series.

(Dover Publications, Inc., 31 East Second St., Mineola, NY 11501.)

Bernath, Stefen. *The Cactus Coloring Book:* saguaro, Bisbee beehive.

Bernath, Stefen. *Common Weeds Coloring Book:* mullein, St.-John's-wort, tansy, yarrow.

Bernath, Stefen. *Garden Flower Coloring Book:* bleeding heart, pansy.

Bernath, Stefen. *House Plants Coloring Book:* aloe vera, fuchsia.

Bernath, Stefen. Ready-to-Use *Floral Spot Illustrations:* sunflower.

Bernath, Stefen. *Trees of the Northeast Coloring Book:* dogwood, oak, pine.

Gaber, Susan. *Treasury of Flower Designs:* peony and floral borders.

Grafton, Carol Berlanger. *1,001 Floral Motifs and Ornaments for Artists:* borders.

Kennedy, Paul E. *American Wildflowers Coloring Book:* black-eyed Susan, buttercup, iris.

Spencer, Edwin Rollin. *All About Weeds:* self-heal.

Tarbox, Charlene. *Floral Designs and Motifs for Artists:* lotus, shooting star, and floral borders.

Please note: The material in this book is meant for reference only and is not intended to treat, diagnose, or prescribe. This information is not a substitute for a consultation with a qualified health care professional or psychotherapist.

CONTENTS

Understanding and dealing with emotions like fear, anger, guilt, resentment, shame, and sadness are a task our society and upbringing give us little assistance with. Flower remedies can help us to understand emotions as they come up and to get free of emotional blocks. Profiles and pictures of Agrimony, Black-eyed Susan, Pine, Sturt Desert Pea, and Willow.

When past events have been painful or traumatic, they tend to leave residues that affect our functioning today. How to recognize shadows of the past; remedies to help release them. Profiles and pictures of Bisbee Beehive Cactus, Centaury, Comfrey, Saguaro, and Star of Bethlehem.

The heart center and its role in relationships. Heart wounds from broken romances and other losses. Flower remedies and other tools for the broken heart and for letting go of lost loves. Essences for couples in conflict. Remedies for sexual wholeness and role conflicts. The dysfunctional family and its effects. Codependency. Profiles and pictures of Bleeding Heart, Dogwood, Heartsease, Peony, and Rhubarb.

Remedies for success in your career, relief of stress, renewed energy, abundance, playfulness, creative self-expression, spiritual development, and an increased capacity for happiness. Profiles and pictures of Iris, Lotus, Oak, Tansy, and Yarrow.

INTRODUCTION

Why is it that flowers are so appealing to us? From earliest times, flowers have enjoyed a special place in our lives, as shown in surviving art, jewelry, crafts, and literature. However, the blooms displayed in paintings, on pottery, and in emblems were not just purely decorative. They also had meanings well known to those who saw them. Through the centuries, a rich, multilayered symbolism grew up around plants, which we will explore throughout this book. People used them to pay homage to the gods and to represent seasons, months, feasts, events, love, and desire. Even the planting of certain flowers, herbs, and trees together had significance. While the symbolism is mostly lost, we still use many flowers and plants in agreement with age-old traditions for holidays, weddings, anniversaries, Valentines, and funerals, without knowing what they mean.

We might say that we love flowers because of their perfume, but, actually, more than 90 percent of flowers have either an unpleasant odor or none at all. So, apart from the pleasurable stimulation of our eyes and sometimes of our noses, why are flowers so universally sought after? They move us very deeply on subtle levels that we do not consciously recognize. Their usefulness as love tokens arises in part from their ability to stimulate the part of the aura corresponding to the heart. In mystical drawings and in meditation, this area is often perceived as a flower. Open blossoms are a gentle, subliminal reminder to the heart to open up and pour out love. The flower children of the Sixties testified to this when they passed out flowers to one another to stimulate a feeling of oneness, and to the police to disarm them and remind them of their humanity.

In this century, flowers are being used in a new and healing way. The essence of the flowers—their energy—is transferred into liquids called flower remedies. These remedies, or essences, are a special yet subtle tool that captures the impact of flowers on our consciousness. Just a few drops of the essences, taken in a regular routine, help us to change unwanted emotional and spiritual patterns. For instance, there are remedies to help release guilt and shame, increase self-esteem, become more open to love, stimulate creativity, and

develop spiritually in a balanced and grounded way. Others can help you learn to deal with your emotions in more mature and conscious ways and to release old shocks and traumas. They are not meant to replace therapy or health care for those who need them. But, as you will learn in chapter 4, the flower remedies can be an excellent adjunct to a variety of healing methods.

Although some early flower remedies were made in the 1500s, their appearance on the modern scene began in the 1930s with Dr. Edward Bach. The Bach remedies are the most well known, but beginning in the 1970s, new companies with new essences came on the scene. While most of the literature focuses solely on the Bach kit, this book will introduce newer remedies from a variety of companies in the United States, Canada, Scotland, and Australia.

The flower remedies found me in 1981. I was at that time rather disillusioned with both of my professions—psychotherapy and astrology. While both produced insight (astrology the faster of the two), neither produced change quickly enough to suit me. Insight without change was frustrating, both for the client and for me as the therapist. I began looking for healing tools to catalyze growth. At that time, I was working with a co-author, Andrew Ramer, who had some interest in herbs. I found a notice about an adult education class on herbology and saved it for Andrew. When he seemed indifferent, I was quite surprised to find myself on the subway, headed for that class.

"Bizarre behavior, old girl," I thought, since physical healing was not at all interesting to me. However, I determinedly went to the class. There seemed to be some reason to be there, and I tend to trust my instincts. In the third session, the teacher introduced the Bach remedies, which continued into the fourth. Their possibilities immediately caught my attention. When that topic was finished, I left the class and started experimenting on my own. "Coincidentally," a co-worker in my social work job, Sherry Mestel, was a Bach practitioner and acted as my mentor in those early days. Soon the remedies proved so helpful that they became an important part of my work and have remained so since then.

I was delighted when Sheila Barry of Sterling Publishing Company asked me to write this book about the flower remedies and their uses. They have been such an important healing tool for my clients—and for me personally—that it is a pleasure to be able to share them with a wider market.

I hope you will find them a similar support in your own quest for self-improvement and for healing for those you care for.

Donna Cunningham
Brooklyn, N.Y. 1992

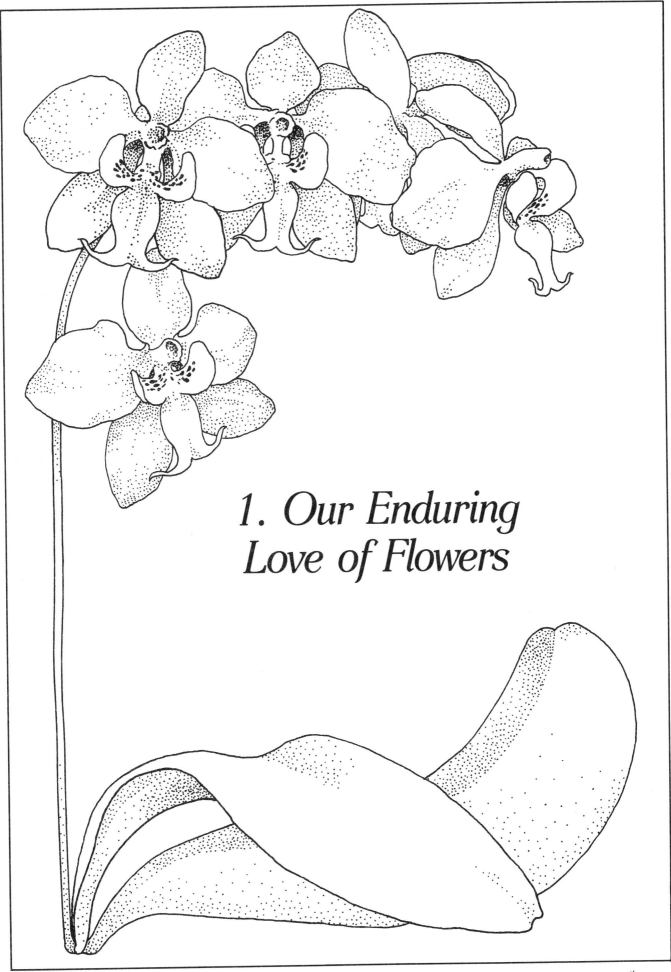

1. Our Enduring Love of Flowers

It's a rare individual who does not enjoy flowers. People love to give them, love to get them, and love to grow them. We celebrate happy times such as weddings and birthdays with them, and take consolation in them in times of illness or grief. In this chapter, we'll look at popular customs that confirm our underlying recognition that flowers have an impact on the human heart. For instance, we'll learn about the Victorians' use of flower language to send messages of love and friendship.

Flower Customs Through the Ages

It is almost instinctive to give your sweetheart flowers in courtship or to patch up a quarrel. When we look through old books and letters, we often find pressed flowers in their pages, preserved as keepsakes. Looking at the dried flowers evokes all the feelings and memories associated with that event. Since bouquets have commonly been a way of declaring love, it's not surprising that many flower customs had to do with romance.

For instance, if lavender thrived in a garden, people believed the daughter of the house would never marry.

To discourage an unwanted suitor, girls gave him a hazel twig, but to encourage him gave birch.

LOVE ORACLES

Many plants were used as love oracles, by which young women would try to divine whom they would marry. At Michaelmas (September 29) girls would gather crab apples and arrange them in the attic to form the initials of their various suitors. Whichever initial was still perfect on Old Michaelmas Day (October 11) was the best choice for a husband. Even today, we use a love oracle when we play the whimsical game of plucking petals off a daisy and counting, "She loves me, she loves me not."

MARRIAGE AND OTHER RITUALS

Once the question of the lucky admirer was settled, flowers were an important part of the marriage ritual. Even now, brides carry a bouquet and toss it to discover which of the single women present will marry next.

Brides wore fragrant honeysuckle wreaths as a symbol of love, constancy, and domestic happiness.

Peach was another favorite for spring brides.

In Mediterranean lands, the bride and groom shared a quince during the wedding to ensure marital happiness and fidelity. Quince is thought to be the fruit Eve gave to Adam, mistranslated into English as the apple.

Today the groom wears a boutonniere, but centuries ago he was given rosemary as a symbol of affectionate remembering. In Hamlet, Ophelia says, "There's rosemary for you: that's for remembrance. I pray you, love, remember."

Rosemary was also placed in coffins and given to those who attended a funeral, so the dead would not be forgotten.

FRIENDSHIP

Loving gestures involving flowers were not limited to sweethearts. For centuries, forget-me-not was given to a friend or loved one as an exhortation to remember the giver. There was a charming tradition wherein friends exchanged these blossoms on Leap Year Day (February 29).

SPECIAL DAYS

The tendency to designate flowers as symbols for special occasions isn't limited to our ancestors. Mother's Day officially began in the United States in 1914. It quickly became the custom for daughters to wear a carnation to church on Mother's Day—red if the mother was still alive, white if she was not. Shamrocks are still used on St.

Patrick's Day, poinsettias around Christmas, and Easter lilies in the spring.

MAGICAL USES

In almost all traditions, including early to medieval Christianity, certain plants were thought to have magical uses.

Druids held red clover in great regard as a charm against evil spirits. In later times, people considered it potent against witches and fairies.

Pennyroyal was said to give protection against the evil eye.

The Chinese used yarrow sticks for divination, through the ancient and wise I Ching.

Witches still use wreaths and dishes of yarrow to clear negativity from the house.

Native American shamans—and their New Age disciples—burn sagebrush to dispel inharmonious energy.

OMENS/TRADITIONS

Like many white flowers, white lilacs were associated with death, and a five-petalled lilac blossom was considered an especially bad omen.

Willows, especially the weeping kind, were a symbol of mourning.

Because people believed deeply in the sympathy between plants and mankind, favorite plants were told when there was a death in the household and bits of black crepe were hung on them. Otherwise, it was feared the plant would wither and die.

Today, we still send floral tributes to funerals.

We have forgotten the reasons for many of these traditions, yet we continue to honor them. In Roman times, holly was an emblem of goodwill, sent as a gift during the feast of Saturn—December 17 to 19. We still decorate with holly during that season.

We also decorate using the mistletoe sacred to ancient Druids for December.

The olive branch was a symbol of peace to the ancient Greeks and is still so viewed today. However, meanings can differ according to the culture. To the Hebrews, the olive branch represented safe travel, because the dove brought it back to the ark after the floods retreated.

Over the ages, poets, legends, fashions at royal courts, and religions added layers of meaning to each flower. For instance, the poppy is an old symbol in many cultures, East and West. However, for the Western world after World War I, it became a widespread tribute to the war dead. The association began because of a song written by a soldier, John McCrae, about poppies growing between rows of graves in Flanders fields. Since 1921, paper poppies have been sold on Memorial Day or its equivalent, in the United Kingdom, the United States, and Canada to support the widows and children of the war dead and, more recently, to benefit the veterans of foreign wars.

The Language of Flowers

One of the most romantic customs was based on the "language of flowers," in which a mixed bouquet might convey a complex message. Used mostly in courtship, it also showed love and admiration between friends and family members. The "language" originated in Japan and China and was adopted in Europe when trade exposed the West to the Oriental cultural influence. Flower language was immensely popular among the nobility during the Middle Ages. In his fascinating book

The Lore of Flowers, Neil Ewart suggests that this was because lords and ladies didn't know how to read and write.[1] It is more gracious to think, however, that in their idle pursuit of pleasure, they escalated romance and intrigue to an art form.

The language of flowers was very prominent in France, where gentlemen might send bouquets to their ladies three or four times a week. It was also the rage in Great Britain during the Tudor period. Shakespeare used it often, to suggest meanings to an audience familiar with their significance. For instance, the pansy was said to be a love potion, and Shakespeare blames pansies for Titania's falling in love with an ass in *A Midsummer Night's Dream*.

If a girl wore a cornflower, she was available for marriage. If a man wore one in his pocket, it showed he was in love.

A woman given a camellia was being told she was "perfected loveliness."

Peach blossoms were a romantic way of saying, "I am your captive."

Morning glory was a token of affection.

Sweet pea meant "Remember me."

The thought behind the bright pink flower known as "shooting star" was "You are my divinity."

A bunch of daisies carried the message "I share your sentiments."

The colors of flowers added nuances and sometimes even conveyed an opposite meaning. The rose was a much-valued token of esteem in early Persia and in Rome, even as it is today. The red rose was a declaration of love. White roses meant "I am worthy of you." Red and white together were a symbol of unity. Yellow roses signified jealousy. A dried rose was a poignant symbol that love was over.

Red chrysanthemums also said "I love you," white meant truth, and yellow portrayed dejection and slighted love.

(In nature, the three most common colors of flowers are white, blue, and red, in that order.)

Flowers as Religious Symbols

There seems to be an almost universal sense of the spiritual nature of flowers and an urge to use them in ceremonies, consecrating them to the divine. Even the poorest church still has a bouquet on the altar on Sunday.

The lotus has been sacred to a variety of faiths for over 5,000 years. In ancient Egypt, it was a reminder of the goal of personal resurrection. Several Eastern religions encourage meditation on the thousand-petalled lotus. Another plant with strong religious meaning is the bo tree. Buddhists revered it because Buddha sat under it in his search for enlightenment.

Sunflowers were unknown to Western culture until Pizarro discovered them in Peru in the 1500s. There the Incas venerated the sunflower as an emblem of their sun god. Priestesses wore large blossoms, hammered of pure gold, on their breasts.

Druids in the British Isles lit fires of gorse at the all-important spring equinox festivals to awaken the young sun.

The shamrock was sacred to the Druids in Ireland long before A.D. 432, when St. Patrick used it to teach about the Trinity. Even today, the shamrock is associated with the Irish and commemorates St. Patrick's Day.

For centuries, the pomegranate, with all its seeds, has been a Mideastern symbol of the Goddess and of fecundity. Women who wanted to know how many children they would have threw a pomegranate to the ground with all their might. They believed that the number of offspring would be shown by the number of seeds that fell out.

The fig was holy to the Hebrews and was later adopted by early Christians because Jesus hungered for them on his way to Bethany.

For both the Hebrews and early Christians, hyssop denoted humility, purification, and cleanliness.

The Easter lily represents purity, chastity, and resurrection.

Many plants were originally named by priests and nuns in the old cloisters, especially those whose duties included gardening. Not only were these clerics better educated than the average person, but they may also have been more attuned to the true meanings of plants through their devotion to prayer and meditation. Many of the names reflect this religious orientation.

Marigold means Mary's Gold, and flowers, especially the white ones, with the word "lady" in their names, were dedicated to Our Lady.

Flowers named Old Man's, however, were thought to belong to the devil.

Religious allusions and moral precepts abounded in tales told about plants. For instance, it was popularly taught that the cross was made of aspen, and thus the tree trembles with shame and horror.

Flower Calendars and Birthday Flowers

Japan and China are flower-conscious cultures, rich in lore and legends reaching far back in time. The Japanese still venerate the ancient art of flower arrangement called ikebana as a form of meditation, in which discerning the proper placement of all the blossoms can take an hour or more. Not only does each blossom in these striking arrangements have meaning, so do the spacing, number, color, and placement. Both the Chinese and Japanese based a calendar on the flower of the month. For instance, the Japanese assigned pine to January, iris to May, peony to June, and willow to November. The oldest and still most popular card game played in Japan has twelve suits to represent the months of this calendar.

In the Middle Ages, as trade was established and the Western world began to have contact with the Orient, it was captivated by floral symbolism and borrowed many Eastern ideas. The Europeans also adopted a calendar that had a flower of the month, but used more familiar varieties. January's flower was the snowdrop, February's was primrose, March claimed violet, and April's emblem was daisy. May was assigned the hawthorn, June the romantic honeysuckle. July's was the water lily, and August's was the poppy. September's flower was morning glory, October was assigned hop, November chrysanthemum, and December holly.

The European calendar evolved into a more elaborate system. Each day of the year was assigned a plant, often for reasons connected with legends and religious tales. Each person had a birthday flower, with all the symbolism attached to that particular plant. In those days, many girls were given names like Violet, Pansy, and Hyacinth, often in accordance with their date of birth. The complete birthday calendar is shown on pages 14–17. (Later, when you learn about the flower remedies, you might want to test the one for your birthday, just to see if it has any special significance for you).

BIRTHDAY FLOWERS

Day	January Flower	Day	February Flower	Day	March Flower
1	oak geranium	1	sweet pea* 4	1	heliotrope
2	multiflora rose	2	yellow rose* 5	2	thorn
3	cactus	3	saffron	3	red pink
4	aloe* 4	4	pansy* 4	4	rose geranium
5	hydrangea	5	marshmallow	5	holly* 1
6	ice plant	6	mistletoe* 3	6	dogbane
7	Japanese rose	7	linden	7	hyacinth* 3
8	laburnum	8	pineapple* 3	8	olive* 1
9	lavender* 2	9	leek	9	anemone* 5
10	withered leaf	10	hawthorn* 3, 6	10	marshmallow#
11	lemon* 4	11	cypress	11	blue violet
12	lemon blossom* 4	12	dew plant	12	maple* 3
13	imperial lily	13	clematis* 1	13	ivy
14	hyssop* 2	14	carnation#* 3	14	white violet
15	marigold* 4	15	hemlock* 7	15	walnut* 1
16	yarrow* 4	16	moss	16	valerian* 3
17	rosemary* 4	17	pea* 7	17	sorrel
18	rue* 4	18	rye grass	18	shamrock
19	sage* 2	19	spruce* 4	19	cohosh#* 4
20	snowdrop* 6	20	yew	20	lettuce
21	southernwood	21	veronica	21	pine* 1
22	mullein* 4	22	amaryllis* 3	22	maidenhair
23	nightshade	23	tansy* 4	23	woodbine
24	oak* 1	24	straw	24	fern
25	motherwort* 3	25	spearmint	25	allspice* 3
26	orange blossom* 4	26	lady's delight	26	pitch pine
27	burning nettle	27	bachelor button* 3	27	fir
28	narcissus* 5	28	calla lily* 2	28	sweetbriar
29	liverwort* 2	29	grass	29	elder* 6
30	mignonette			30	horehound* 3
31	periwinkle* 5, 3			31	love-lies-bleeding

Where there is a #, a more modern name has been substituted. The symbol * indicates that the flower remedy exists. Companies offering the remedy are shown by the number after the *, as follows: 1 = Bach, 2 = FES, 3 = Pegasus, 4 = both FES and Pegasus, 5 = Petite Fleur, 6 = Harebell, 7 = Other. See Appendix A. Other companies may offer these remedies as well.

FROM AN OLD TRADITION

April

Day	Flower
1	columbine* 4
2	rush
3	meadow saffron
4	reed
5	mouse-ear chickweed* 6
6	myrrh
7	hop* 4
8	almond tree* 3
9	balsam
10	barberry
11	beech* 1
12	bindweed* 6
13	cinquefoil* 2
14	birch* 4
15	china aster
16	crocus blossom
17	daisy* 6
18	wild grape
19	honey flower
20	withered rose
21	honeysuckle* 1
22	yellow jasmine* 2
23	lady's slipper* 3
24	musk plant
25	peach blossom* 4
26	bridal rose
27	broken straw
28	yellow violet
29	wormwood* 3
30	vernal grass

May

Day	Flower
1	American aster#
2	chickweed* 3
3	May rose
4	myrtle
5	ophrys
6	quince* 2
7	primrose* 5
8	white poppy
9	snowball
10	red poppy* 6
11	sensitive plant* 4
12	Star of Bethlehem* 1
13	strawberry* 4
14	sumac
15	sweet William
16	syringa (lilac)* 3
17	thistle* 6
18	vervain* 1
19	trillium#* 2
20	wallflower* 4
21	weeping willow
22	willow* 1
23	water lily
24	aconite#* 3
25	rhubarb* 6
26	phlox* 3
27	meadowsweet* 6, 3
28	oleander* 4
29	French marigold* 3
30	Carolina rose
31	pink

June

Day	Flower
1	marjoram* 6
2	double red pink
3	yellow pink
4	daily rose
5	Lancaster rose
6	thornapple
7	red tulip* 6
8	variegated tulip
9	thyme* 4
10	pomegranate* 3
11	black poplar
12	prickly pear
13	potato blossom* 3
14	mountain pink
15	wild plum
16	fly orchis
17	palm
18	mustard seed* 1
19	mulberry tree* 3
20	black mulberry
21	peony* 4
22	passionflower* 4
23	pasqueflower* 3
24	hemp
25	hollyhock* 4
26	sweet scabious
27	schinus
28	snapdragon* 4
29	St.-John's-Wort* 4
30	sunflower* 4

Note: Material on birth dates is adapted from Jobes, Gertrude, *Dictionary of Mythology, Folklore, and Symbols*, New York: Scarecrow Press, 1962, pp. 214 to 217, and is reprinted with the publisher's permission.

BIRTHDAY FLOWERS

July

Day	Flower
1	sycamore* 3
2	xanthium
3	wood sorrel
4	water willow
5	crown of roses
6	white rosebud* 6
7	red rosebud* 6
8	white rose* 6
9	wild rose#* 1
10	fig tree* 4
11	angelica* 4
12	basil* 4
13	daffodil#* 2
14	bay
15	belladonna* 3
16	harebell#* 6
17	bilberry
18	bittersweet* 4
19	blackberry#* 4
20	bulrush
21	Canterbury bell
22	celandine* 3
23	Indian plum
24	white lilac
25	lilac* 4
26	magnolia* 5
27	saxifrage#
28	money plant#* 3 (honesty)#* 6
29	verbena* 5
30	Patagonian mint
31	osier (a willow)

August

Day	Flower
1	Burgundy rose
2	damask rose
3	moss rose* 5
4	morning glory* 4
5	hundred-leaved rose
6	sardony
7	saintfoil
8	scabious
9	witch hazel* 3
10	whortleberry
11	fireweed#* 4
12	vine* 1
13	vetch
14	thrift
15	throatwort
16	butterfly orchis
17	pear* 4
18	blue periwinkle
19	pimpernel* 6
20	crow foot
21	cuckoo flower
22	currant* 6
23	daffodil* 5
24	dahlia* 3
25	sweet flag* 3
26	life everlasting
27	filbert
28	flax
29	flower-of-an-hour
30	flowering reed
31	foxglove* 6

September

Day	Flower
1	fumitory
2	helenium
3	hepatica
4	hoya
5	mimosa
6	iris* 4
7	lily of the valley
8	madder
9	monkshood* 4
10	tear drop
11	cranberry* 3
12	jonquil
13	love-in-a-snail
14	acacia* 3
15	rose acacia
16	adonis
17	box
18	buttercup* 4
19	cabbage* 3
20	China pink
21	corn* 4
22	primrose#
23	ivy sprig
24	cress
25	crocus* 7
26	dock
27	dandelion* 2
28	gooseberry* 3
29	guelder rose
30	bluebell* 6

Where there is a #, a more modern name has been substituted. The symbol * indicates that the flower remedy exists. Companies offering the remedy are shown by the number after the *, as follows: 1 = Bach, 2 = FES, 3 = Pegasus, 4 = both FES and Pegasus, 5 = Petite Fleur, 6 = Harebell, 7 = Other. See Appendix A. Other companies may offer these remedies as well.

FROM AN OLD TRADITION

October

Day	Flower
1	horse chestnut* 1
2	juniper
3	wheat
4	Venus's looking glass
5	turnip
6	tuberose* 3
7	traveler's joy
8	tamarisk
9	celandine#* 3
10	stock* 5
11	black-eyed Susan* 4
12	mundi rose
13	red rose* 6
14	China rose
15	raspberry* 3
16	split reed
17	single reed
18	rhododendron* 3
19	Austrian rose
20	rose campion* 5
21	buttercup#* 2
22	red primrose
23	polyanthus* 7
24	plane tree
25	Indian pink* 2
26	larch* 1
27	peppermint* 4
28	osmunda
29	oxeye daisy
30	parsley
31	common nettle* 6

November

Day	Flower
1	nasturtium* 4, 6
2	mountain ash
3	mugwort* 2, 6
4	mushroom* 5
5	mimosa
6	mandrake* 3
7	marvel of Peru
8	lupine
9	lotus flower* 4
10	lotus* 4
11	lotus tree
12	linchen
13	field lily
14	yellow lily
15	laurestine
16	mountain laurel
17	laurel
18	houstonia
19	hornbeam* 1
20	honeysuckle* 1
21	hawkweed* 6
22	gourd
23	fuchsia* 4
24	dark geranium
25	nutmeg geranium
26	silver leaf geranium
27	gentian* 1
28	gorse* 1
29	goldilocks
30	goldenrod* 4

December

Day	Flower
1	scarlet geranium
2	teasel (#boneset)
3	French willow
4	flower de luce
5	fennel* 3
6	dragon plant
7	diomosa
8	althea (hollyhock)
9	creeper
10	coronilla
11	cockle
12	coriander* 4
13	citron
14	coxcomb
15	coreopsis* 2
16	rock rose* 1
17	chamomile* 2
18	cedar of Lebanon
19	carnation
20	cardinal flower
21	japonica
22	petunia* 4
23	bear's-breech
24	chrysanthemum* 2
25	Christmas rose (helleborus* 3)
26	balm of Gilead* 3
27	ash tree
28	arbor vitae (tree of life* 3)
29	amaranthus* 3
30	ambrosia
31	apple blossom* 2

Note: Material on birth dates is adapted from Jobes, Gertrude, *Dictionary of Mythology, Folklore, and Symbols*, New York: Scarecrow Press, 1962, pp. 214 to 217, and is reprinted with the publisher's permission.

What Tree Were You Born Under?

Can you imagine someone coming up to you at a cocktail party and asking, "What tree are you?" The ancient Druids may have done just that at their get-togethers, which would doubtless have made our happy hours pale by comparison! Cultures all around the world spontaneously developed their own brand of astrology, and these early inhabitants of the British Isles had one based on trees, which were sacred to them and which they believed were inhabited by nature spirits. These trees were part of an elaborate system of seasonal magic and divination, based on an eighteen-letter alphabet with a tree assigned to each letter.[2] So that you'll know the answer if someone asks you your tree, here they are.

Season	Birth Tree	Season	Birth Tree
New Year	Silver fir, elm	Autumn Equinox	Aspen
Spring Equinox	Broom	Winter Solstice	Yew
Summer Solstice	Heather		

Date	Birth Tree	Date	Birth Tree
December 23	Mistletoe	6/11 to 7/8	Oak
12/24 to 1/21	Birch	7/9 to 8/5	Holly or gorse
1/22 to 2/18	Rowan	8/6 to 9/2	Hazel
2/19 to 3/18	Ash	9/3 to 9/30	Vine
3/19 to 4/15	Alder	10/1 to 10/28	Ivy
4/16 to 5/13	Willow	10/29 to 11/25	Reed, dwarf elder
5/14 to 6/10	White thorn	11/26 to 12/22	Elder

We don't have space here to give a reading of your birth tree, but a delightful book and set of cards by Liz and Colin Murray, based on these ancient symbols, are available in many New Age bookstores. The book is called *The Celtic Tree Oracle*. Llewellyn's *Celtic Magic*, by D. J. Conway, is also an excellent source of information.

Astrology and Flowers

My French informants tell me that their national motto is "Why do it simply when you can make it complicated?" That seems to be borne out of an old Gallic form of astrology in which your birth sign is a plant. Each of the 73 signs covered five consecutive days, with personality traits and lucky days attributed to natives of that sign. My knowledge of the system is limited to a set of postcards encountered in a French seaside resort—alas! all in French. (I am an ivy, though, and that felt right!) Astrological contacts in France don't seem to know much about the system.

Flower Emblems of the Signs

Sign	Flower	Sign	Flower
Aries	violet	Libra	morning glory
Taurus	daisy	Scorpio	hop
Gemini	hawthorn	Sagittarius	chrysanthemum
Cancer	honeysuckle	Capricorn	holly
Leo	water lily	Aquarius	snowdrop
Virgo	hazel	Pisces	primrose.[3]

What Your Own Favorite Flowers Tell About You

For all our education and sophistication, we know little about floral messages today. Innuendos that delighted Shakespeare's audiences pass right over our heads, even those of us who are Shakespeare lovers. Someone could send us a thoroughly insulting bouquet and we'd never catch on! When it comes to flowers, we are reduced to the status of the untutored individual who attends an art exhibit and says, "I know what I like."

We know what we like, all right, even if we don't know why. Our personal favorites say a great deal about us, as you'll come to understand in the course of this book. We are drawn to certain plants and repelled by others. These reactions arise from deeper levels of being—the universal and collective levels where floral symbolism still operates.

As we study flower essences and their meanings in the chapters that follow, we will gain greater understanding of these likes and dislikes. You may already be able to make some guesses.

A little girl whose father had gone to war and whose beloved grandfather had died often sat for hours under a weeping willow. She had no idea this tree was a symbol for mourning, yet she felt comforted. When she began using flower essences, still not aware of the symbolism, she had to take Willow essence for many months.

Plants you detest may tell just as much as your favorites.

Peonies repelled one woman, seemingly because of the ants that crawl in their petals. She was embarrassed to find out that in the language of flowers, peonies represent shame.

Flower essence practitioner Alexis Rotella says that the flowers we grew up around, especially those we loved as children, have special importance and strong healing power for us. My suspicion is that the plants weren't there by accident. Your parents or grandparents doubtless were drawn to them because of some dim awareness of their healing properties for certain family patterns, which were passed down to you. Think back and remember what those flowers were, especially the ones with sentimental value, and notice their meaning as we go along. Later in the book, you may want to see whether flower essences made from them might be good for you.

As an example, one young woman, an only child born to older parents, had lost most of the adults in her family by the time she was 25. She yearned for her family, whom she had loved dearly, and often felt alone in life, even though she had good friends. Whenever she saw a honeysuckle vine, she would well up with tears, recalling that this vine had been in her grandmother's back yard when she was a child. The flower remedy Honeysuckle is for nostalgia and a feeling that the past was better. After she took it for a few months, the feeling of being alone in life had receded, and she felt more resolved about her losses.

Why Do We Assign Meanings to Flowers?

It is mysterious, isn't it, why cultures of all ages, all over the world, attribute meaning to flowers. Why would a rose represent love—why shouldn't a chair or an egg be just as symbolic of love? Why should an Easter lily represent resurrection when a barn door does not? Let's look at some possible answers to these questions. It is not necessary for you to accept any of these ideas in order to work with this book. However, they do provide some interesting theories about how the ancient and universal trait of attributing meaning to flowers came into being.

All symbolism derives from conscious and unconscious associations between one thing and another, and floral symbolism is no different. In the 1500s, a master physician and herbalist called Paracelsus elucidated the doctrine of signatures. He and many others of the time believed that the shape, color, taste, smell, and other properties of a plant gave hints of its use in healing. For instance, he observed that the leaf of an herb used to treat the liver was in fact shaped like the liver. The leaf of the cyclamen is shaped and marked like an ear, and it was thought effective in dealing with diseases of that organ.

As an example of this work, Paracelsus observed that Christmas rose (*Helleborus niger*) bloomed in winter and concluded that it had rejuvenative powers. He introduced the plant into the pharmacopeia of the time and recommended it for people over fifty. Later, it was found that this plant did have an effect on arteriosclerosis.[4]

Another widely held theory of the time was that whenever an illness was found in a particular location, plants growing in the area would heal it. For example, willow was thought to be good for rheumatoid arthritis because it grew in damp places, and this type of arthritis is made worse by the damp. Later, an extract of the bark was used to make aspirin, a primary drug for arthritis.

Some flower essence practitioners have taken this concept to mean that we should primarily use the essences of flowers growing in our own area. The fallacy in this is that, as worldwide travel began from the 1500s onward, plants from any given area have spread throughout the world, wherever growing conditions permit. A plant growing as a giant jungle shrub in Brazil may be available as a mini-houseplant in Alaska.

Modern botanists reject the doctrine of signatures just as modern doctors tend to reject the healing properties of herbs. However, both herbalists and flower essence practitioners continue to find helpful hints in such connections. Whether or not you find them a key to healing, no doubt you can see that symbolism can derive from associations like these. For instance, it's not hard to understand why Hawaiians regarded the banana as a fertility symbol and why the peach has been used to represent the female. We will refer back to this doctrine of signatures from time to time, as it is often a way to grasp and remember the meaning of a flower essence.

The Belief in Plant Angels or Spirits

We've seen that it is nearly universal to associate flowers with spirituality, no matter what your particular faith may be. Students of meditation may be taught to gaze at a single bloom and empty their minds. Why should this practice uplift us spiritually? One theory held by mystics and meditators over the ages is that there are spiritual forces associated with every species of plant. These angels or beings of light, known as devas, are responsible for co-creating the plant along with the Divine and for maintaining its growth.

This same idea seems to have developed spontaneously in many parts of the world. The traditional May Day celebrations and dances around the maypole in the British Isles and its colonies were originally serious pagan rituals honoring the spirits of trees. Long before explorers came to the Americas, Native Americans believed profoundly in the holy aliveness of the earth and the plant kingdom. They would not pick a plant without asking its permission and would leave behind a gift, usually cornmeal or tobacco. Even today, their ceremonies before cutting a tree are lengthy ones, in which they pray to be worthy to take the life of that tree.

All over the world, native peoples seem to revere plant spirits, especially those of trees. Tribesman of central Africa believe that if a tree is cut down, the spirit in it may become so angry that it will cause the chief and his family to die. To prevent this, the person who is chopping down the tree will first make a cut and suck some of the sap. This makes him a blood brother of the tree, which entitles him to cut it down.

George Washington Carver, the great agricultural chemist who was born a slave, revolutionized the economy of the South when he discovered hundreds of uses for the peanut and other southern plants. He made no secret of the fact that he communicated with plants and asked them questions about their uses. He said, "All flowers talk to me, and so do hundreds of little living things in the woods. I learn what I know by watching and loving everything."[5] It is entirely possible that Carver was talking to the plant angels, rather than the plants.

It is not well known that Luther Burbank, the horticulturist who developed over 2000 distinct species of plants, was a mystic. He was strongly telepathic, consulted spiritualists, was a friend of the famous yogi Paramahansa Yogananda, and was able to heal by the laying on of hands. Burbank believed that plants adapt themselves to human wishes. In initiating new species, he formed mental images of the results he desired, with great success. For instance, he wanted to breed a form of spineless cactus. He felt the spines were protection against predators and that cacti growing in an atmosphere of love would not need spines. So he talked to them. He told them they had nothing to fear, that they didn't need their thorns, as he would protect them. With this communication and the mental image of what he wanted, he successfully produced a species without thorns.[6]

A more modern case in point is the work at Findhorn in Scotland. The landscape in the area is a near-desert of sand and gravel. Although neighbors seem to have limited success with their gardening efforts, the Findhorn gardens are lushly green, with huge vegetables. The difference is that the people who live at Findhorn consciously and consistently work in cooperation with the devas, invoking them and thanking them as they work. Rich gardens where nothing at all should grow are the result.

There are many people like Carver, Burbank, and the Findhorn gardeners who receive messages from plants through meditation and conscious attunement. In particular, the great majority of people who make flower remedies from scratch, and many remedy practitioners, find attuning to the flowers both satisfying and helpful. People who love working with plants but who have no conscious belief in this level of spirit could also become attuned to plant angels. They might use this psychic connection to make flowers and crops grow better.

Do Plants Have Consciousness?

There is also evidence to suggest that individual plants themselves have consciousness. If you find that an outrageous notion, consider the experiments done by lie detector expert Cleve Backster in the 1960s. He carried on a wide variety of tests in which the plants were hooked up to a specialized polygraph. His experiments showed that the plants had strong reactions to a variety of threats. These reactions were similar to what humans would show on polygraph examinations under severe emotional stress. For instance, he had only to think strongly about setting fire to a leaf, without making a move, and the plant would register a dramatic response.

In one experiment, a "killer" was chosen from six college students by lot. No one but the killer knew who was chosen—not even Backster. The culprit went into the lab secretly that night and destroyed a plant in front of another plant. The next morning, the six students were marched by the "witness" plant, one by one. There was no reaction to the innocent students. When the student who had actually destroyed the plant passed by, the witness plant reacted strongly.

In another instance, three plants attached to polygraphs were placed in separate rooms. In still another room, a machine was programmed to dump live brine shrimp into boiling water at varied intervals. Polygraphs of all three plants registered strong emotional reactions each time the shrimp hit the water and died. Thus, it could be concluded that not only are plants apparently connected and concerned about each other, they are concerned about the animal kingdom as well.[7]

Most startling of all, the experiments by Backster and the people who followed in his footsteps in the early 1970s seemed to prove that plants were especially concerned about and connected to human beings. When Backster was away on a trip, the plants often reacted positively as he got on the plane to come home. At one point, Backster accidentally cut himself, and the plants registered alarm. So, the old tradition of plants being notified and draped in mourning when a member of the household died may not be so naive after all.

There are many strange phenomena to suggest that being a vegetable doesn't mean you don't have consciousness. Perhaps we're going to have to quit using the word vegetable as a derogatory term! If you wanted to know more about these and other fascinating experiments, the best source is *The Secret Life of Plants* by Peter Tompkins and Christopher Bird.

What We Can Learn from Our Ancestors

Maybe our ancestors couldn't read books, but they could read flowers and plants. Their senses weren't bombarded with television, newspapers, and other media, so they could more readily tune in to messages from nature. We can read, but we are the equivalent of dyslexic when it comes to the meanings and symbolism of the flowers— dysfloric, perhaps?

If you want to know more about floral meanings and legends, you may wish to read books on flower lore. The ones in the Bibliography are excellent, but some are no longer in print. The two that are currently most available and most fascinating are Josephine Addison's *The Illustrated Plant Lore*[8] and Sheila Pickles's beautifully boxed and perfumed *The Language of Flowers*, in itself a pleasurable token for someone you love.[9] Currently available and rich with lore are two herbals: Paul Beyerl's *The Master Book of Herbalism*, and Scott Cunningham's *Cunningham's Encyclopedia of Magical Herbs*, both listed in the Bibliography. (I know you're asking, and, no, we're not related.)

Studying ancient meanings of plants is not just quaint and interesting, it is a way to regain lost knowledge and get back in communication with the plant kingdom, on which our lives depend. The more out of touch with nature we are, the more destructive we are to our environment. If we hadn't lost our habit of respectful listening to plants, we wouldn't be altering the atmosphere irrevocably by bulldozing the rain forests. Even home gardeners, if they hadn't lost connection with the plants they raise, wouldn't be poisoning the land by using weed killers rather than better informed means.

The other consequence of getting out of touch is that we've forgotten how to heal ourselves naturally. In the chapters that follow, we'll learn about a natural system of healing based on flowers—the flower remedies.

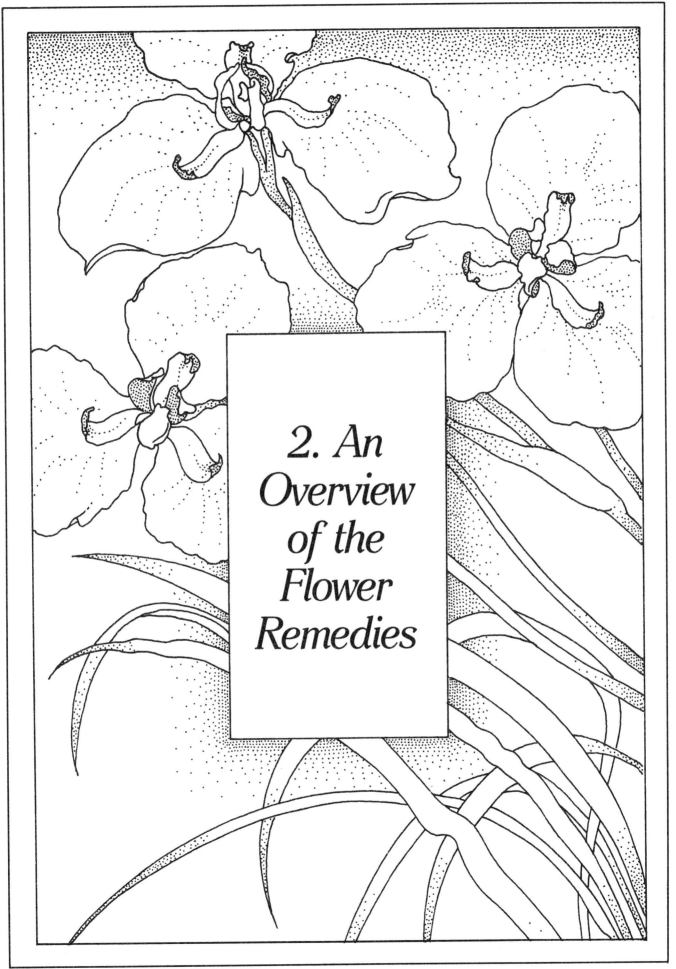

2. An Overview of the Flower Remedies

Those who love flowers and sense their healing effects may feel an instinctive and joyful connection to the flower remedies. They are also called flower essences; the two terms are used interchangeably.

These mild, natural substances represent a well-tested but nontraditional healing system that works gently on the mind/body connection. They are liquids you take under the tongue. Don't confuse them with aromatherapy, in which you inhale the perfume of the plant. Flower remedies have no aroma of their own. While not a substitute for psychotherapy or health care for those who need them, essences are a useful adjunct to therapy, healing, or self-improvement efforts. They can help us become whole by releasing past conditioning and accumulations of negative emotions.

How Essences Help Change Unwanted Thought Patterns

While medicines and herbs have an impact primarily on the physical body, flower remedies affect emotional and spiritual well-being. They are a subtle but powerful way of changing consciousness, even deeply ingrained thought patterns. Thoughts have great power; they create the reality we live in. Recurrent ideas and deep convictions attract people and conditions that recreate what we believe to be true about life, ourselves, and other people. Many of you work with visualizations to change consciousness. Visualizations have proved very powerful—even affecting the immune system. This was demonstrated by cancer patients under the supervision of the Simontons, who successfully used visualizations to strengthen the immune system.[1]

Flower remedies also work well with affirmations and other consciousness-changing techniques such as psychotherapy or Neurolinguistic Programming (NLP), a blend of techniques used by the world's best therapists. Because the essences work on deeper levels of thought and beliefs, they enhance the success of tools that work on consciousness.

For vast numbers of people, thoughts and attitudes are what make us happy or unhappy. One person in a particular job may be contented and fulfilled, while another feels frustrated, resentful, and even demeaned by the very same set of tasks. The differences are in attitudes and past conditioning, rather than in circumstances.

Even if you are in a realistically difficult or painful situation, the remedies can lend a new perspective. You can come to view the past differently, release burdensome accumulations of stress, fatigue, or painful emotions, and gain new strength and hope.

Erroneous conclusions or negative recurrent thoughts make life more difficult even in the best of times. A poor self-concept is no more than a habit of thinking disparagingly of yourself, but it can retard your progress as if a ball and chain were attached to your leg. Flower remedies, like the ones that are recommended for self-esteem, support us in changing self-destructive beliefs that make us miserable. When beliefs and attitudes change, very often the conditions around us change, too.

Breaking Unwanted Emotional Habits

As we go along, many unpleasant emotions will be revealed as no more than bad habits, however deeply entrenched. Flower remedies enable us to recognize and break these habits. For instance, they help us change an overattachment to either the future or the past—the kind of attachment that makes it hard for us to live fully today.

Guilt and resentment are a well-entwined pair of emotions that estrange us from ourselves and others. These feelings aren't facts, but mental and emotional habits of reliving past events.

Pine and Crab Apple, by Bach Company, are two remedies related to guilt, and their Willow and Holly are related to resentment.

Throughout this book, the names of remedies will be capitalized to distinguish them from the plant or herb of the same name. For example, willow refers to the tree itself and Willow to the remedy.

Worry, fear, and anxiety are also undesirable emotional habits. Unless we are in actual danger, when they help to provide necessary caution and information, these emotions result from rehearsing the future in a negative light. Since we can control neither the past nor the future, emotional habits like these drain us needlessly and keep us from functioning as well as we possibly can right now. A large number of remedies for fear are available from various companies.

When you take a remedy, notice how your reactions change. At first, it seems that you're more conscious of what you're thinking. This new awareness may be surprising and even uncomfortable, because you've been so unconscious of your reactions in the past. As you continue to take the drops, these responses start to seem ridiculous. Finally, you're ready to let go of them—maybe even laugh at them!

The essences are not a magic cure-all and not a medication like a tranquilizer. They are not a way to avoid feelings—though they promote working through them more quickly and profoundly. In our feel-good society, many people don't like the work involved in getting well. They are looking for a magic potion or pill to take all their troubles away. The process initiated by flower remedies requires work and time, like any other healing tool. You can't just take one dose and change into a saint or be divinely happy forever after. Sorry!

You may need to take a particular remedy for months when you tackle a deeply ingrained pattern. If you're working toward self-improvement already, you'll undoubtedly still need your therapist, health care practitioner, or support group. But, if you use the remedies consistently, you may find that emotional backlogs clear out much more quickly, and you experience a great deal more clarity than you did before.

One of my clients, a young man, was recovering from a troubled adolescence of drug and alcohol abuse. He had been sober and drug free for several years through A.A. and was also in therapy. One of his difficulties in sobriety was that he went through lists in his mind all day long. It was a form of mental torture that nothing, including prayer, had overcome. I gave him a bottle of White Chestnut, the Bach remedy for worries and unwanted thoughts. No result. I gave him a second bottle. No result. A third—no result. I was ready to conclude that something had gone wrong with his wiring from all those drugs. He, being a good obsessive, was willing to take a fourth bottle. When he finished it, the list-making abruptly ceased and has not returned in over five years. It is unusual to have to take so many bottles before seeing any improvement, but he was rewarded for persevering.

The Flower Remedies and Health

Flower remedies are *not* herbal extracts, even though some are made from the flowers of such herbs as chamomile, comfrey, goldenseal, and cayenne. Extracts or tinctures contain the actual plant and have potent effects on the body, being prepared specifically for medicinal purposes. Because of their strength, herbs and herbal extracts are not to be taken lightly. In the wrong amount, at the wrong time, using the wrong part of the plant for the wrong person, herbs can be toxic.

Flower remedies, however, are self-adjusting, which means that when the remedy is incorrect, it simply has no effect. There are no harmful side-effects, either. The purpose of a flower remedy is also different from that of herbs. For instance, a cup of chamomile tea can be relaxing after a stressful day, and many people need to unwind almost nightly from their pressured lives. The essence Chamomile, however, when taken over a period of time, allows the individual to make changes so there is less tension to begin with.

The essences are not medications for physical ailments, although they can support physical healing. Their effect is not direct. There is no one remedy, for example, for ulcers, high blood pressure, or menopause. Instead, the mind/body connection becomes involved, and an improved emotional outlook paves the way for an improved physical condition. Traditional physicians are now admitting that stress and crisis have a profound effect on health and that negative emotions can lower our resistance to disease. Dr. Philip M. Chancellor's *Handbook of the Bach Flower Remedies* documents case after case of physical illness improving or clearing up as the underlying emotional difficulties were alleviated through the remedies.[2]

I cannot emphasize too strongly that any serious physical problem requires care and supervision by a qualified and licensed health care practitioner. Since some health practitioners use essences in combination with other methods, you may find one who will work this way. Gregory Vlamis's book, *Flowers to the Rescue*, contains hundreds of case studies submitted by doctors and other health care practitioners.[3] Holistic physicians and practitioners who accept the power of the mind/body connection are generally the most open. Look at listings in your local New Age newspaper, or ask for a referral from one of the flower essence companies.

What the Remedies Are

Having found out what the remedies are *not*, no doubt you're wondering exactly what they *are*. They are the life force of plants collected from the energy field or aura of the plant.

Life force energy is what gives plants, animals, and people their vitality. The existence of energy fields around plants, people, and other living things has been demonstrated by Kirlian photography. You may have seen one picture that shows light glowing around a leaf, while a second, taken after part of the leaf was cut away, shows light still glowing around the whole leaf—even the portion that is no longer there.[4]

In making flower essences, the life force energy of the plant is captured by picking flowers at dawn at the height of their vitality. They are placed in water in the sunlight for several hours. The resulting liquid is enhanced in a variety of ways, diluted and strengthened several times, and then bottled. The essence practitioner picks and mixes remedies suited to your particular concerns. You generally take the mixture four times a day, noticing and reporting your reactions.

Do the Remedies Work?

How do we know the remedies work? The Bach remedies have been clinically tested in Great Britain and the United States for over 50 years. They are derived from the older, alternative medical model of homeopathy, which is well accepted in Europe and is the health care system of the British Royal Family. A great many doctors, chiropractors, psychotherapists, and other health care practitioners all over the world also use the essences.

A well-designed study on the Bach remedies was done by Michael Weisglas for his Ph.D. dissertation, as described in *The Flower Essence Journal*.[5] In what is known technically as a double-blind study, he took three groups of students and gave them a psychological test. One group was given a placebo bottle indistinguishable from the others, but containing no actual flower remedies. The second group had four remedies in the bottle, and the third had seven. The students were retested after three weeks and then again after six weeks. The group with the placebo did not change, but the group with four remedies had very positive, statistically significant changes. (The group with seven remedies had more difficulty.)

Kirlian photographs have been taken of the effects of Vita Florum, a British flower combination that the maker, Elizabeth Bellhouse, calls homeovitic rather than homeopathic. A dramatic series of photographs shows weak light around the hands of a woman before she took Vita Florum. Another, taken immediately after, shows a stronger light that increases in photos taken one minute later and two minutes later. The photo taken after three minutes had passed reveals a brilliant light around the hands.

Another of the Kirlian photographs in the Vita Florum collection shows a weak aura around a drop of tap water, as opposed to a radiant energy around it after the addition of a drop of Vita Florum.[6]

Readers who find these ideas difficult to accept are urged simply to try the remedies and experience the effects personally. A fair test requires only an open mind and careful observations, perhaps keeping a written record or journal of your process. Remember, the students in Dr. Weisglas' study weren't operating on faith. In the end, of course, it is up to you to decide whether the remedies are effective for your own healing process.

Dr. Edward Bach and the Bach Flower Remedies

Flower remedies were known in India and China and to the Australian aboriginals centuries ago. In Europe, they were made in the 1500s by Paracelsus, the master physician and alchemist mentioned earlier. The modern pioneer in the field was Dr. Edward Bach, a well-respected English physician and homeopath who had done important work on immunology. In addition to traditional medicine and homeopathy, there is evidence that he read Paracelsus' writings. In the early 1930s, he left his successful practice and began gathering wildflowers and plants to develop his flower remedies. Those who would like to know more about Dr. Bach and the discovery process for his remedies would be interested in Norah Weeks's *The Medical Discoveries of Edward Bach.*[7]

Since his death, the Bach Centre in England has continued to investigate and document the uses of his remedies through over fifty years of clinical case histories. As a result, these remedies are widely accepted and known in England, in a way they are not in the United States. Part of the difference is that in England and parts of Europe the closely allied science of homeopathy is still well respected, whereas in the United States the American Medical Association was able to suppress it early in this century. The differences between homeopathy and flower essences are too lengthy and complex to go into here. The major differences is that homeopathic remedies are diluted and potentized as many as 200 times, while most flower remedies are potentized only six times. Thus, the more potent homeopathic treatment should be undertaken only with a trained homeopath, while flower remedies can safely be self-chosen and -administered.

The Bach remedies were developed during the Depression era, and various people have noted that they seem to reflect the climate of their time. There are many remedies for depression, discouragement, and fear among the 38 plants in the kit. There is also a strong focus on healing such toxic emotions as resentment, guilt, hate, and the experience of being a victim.

Of all the remedies, the Bach collection is by far the most commonly available. Many health food stores carry them. You may purchase single bottles or the entire kit. You may also order directly from Bach, either the parent company in the United Kingdom or their representatives:

Ellon Bach/USA, Inc.
644 Merrick Road
Lynbrook, NY 11563

Bach Flower Remedies
   Ltd
The Bach Centre
Mt. Vernon, Sotwell
Wallingford, Oxon
   OX10 OPZ
U.K.

Beyond Bach—A View of the Newer Flower Remedies

Dr. Edward Bach's genius and contribution as the father of the flower essences are undeniable. Some of his followers, however, would have us believe his 38 remedies are the only ones possible and his interpretations are carved in stone. In this, they are like the medieval church, which wanted people to believe interpretation was not possible to the layman, and that spiritual revelation ended on the last page of the Bible. In fact, there are a variety of companies around the world making very fine essences, often even more relevant to the concerns of today.

Next to Bach, the best known are undoubtedly the "California Essences." This is a misnomer, of course, because there are several companies making remedies in California, but it refers to the highly regarded line of Flower Essence Services, or FES. Having worked with the Bach essences for many years, the founders of FES, Richard Katz and Patricia Kaminski, wanted to explore the effects of remedies made from North American plant species. After extensive testing with health practitioners, they released their first kit to the public in 1978. They now have a repertory of 72 well-documented essences and hundreds they are continuing to research.

The FES collection, evolving in California during the Human Potential Movement of the 1970s and 1980s, was as much affected by the climate of those times as Bach was by his. Their set includes selections for self-esteem, creativity, and spiritual development. There are several for more loving relationships and even for sexual health. Their brochure, "Flower Essence Therapy," describes their 72 major remedies and is beautifully illustrated.

Research and education are perhaps the distinguishing feature of the work of FES. Co-director Patricia Kaminski says, "Our society warmly and openly receives research and case studies from any and all who wish to contribute." Each spring and summer, FES conducts richly informative certification programs for people who wish to use these essences in their practice. Part of the course is experiential, conducting observations and meditations on the flowers in their native habitats. For a catalog of remedies, aromatic oils, flower photographs, and books, write to the Flower Essence Society, Box 459, Nevada City, CA 95959.

One of the more recently established American companies that deserves special mention is the Alaskan Flower Essence Project. Their flowers and plants are collected in the unspoiled Alaskan wilderness—and they are possibly some of the purest concentrations of pure life force energy anywhere on the planet. Those who are psychically attuned get strong sensations of vitality when holding a bottle of these essences. For information and a catalog, write to the Alaskan Flower Essence Project, P.O. Box 1369, Homer, AK 99603-1369.

At the First International Flower Essence Congress in May 1990, I met the founders of two companies from Australia and acquired their books and some of their essences. Because of the island continent's millennia of isolation, their ancient plant species come from an evolutionary stock entirely different from our own. The flowers themselves, from their pictures, are exotically beautiful. The names alone are fascinating: Southern Cross, Purple Kangaroo Paw, Happy Wanderer, Sunshine Wattle, Illyarrie, Isopogon, Wedding Bush, and Billy Goat Plum.

The essences seem quite powerful. In particular, the Australian Bush Essences' Emergency Formula is impressive. There does seem to be a difference between it and Bach's Rescue Remedy—sometimes one is called for, sometimes the other, sometimes both, but in sequence. They also have a wonderful combination called the Cognis Essence, which greatly enhances learning. When ordering either, specify that you want a stock bottle, because it's usually packaged in the diluted form. (Their prices are given in Australian dollars.) You can write for catalogs to:

Australian Bush
  Flower Essences
Box 531
Spit Junction, NSW
2088 Australia

Living Essences
Box 355
Scarborough,
  W. Australia
6019 Australia

An easy and inexpensive alternative that newcomers in particular find attractive are the premixed combinations that several companies provide. The most generally available of these are by Deva, a California-based company that has been gathering flowers and combining remedies since the early 1970s. Look for them in health food stores, or write to Deva at Natural Labs, Box 229, Encinitas, CA 92024. Among their ready-to-use formulas, which number over 30, are remedies for stress and tension, fatigue, anger and resentment, guilt, worry, depression, change and transition, and grief. I don't use combinations, preferring to individualize the remedies given to clients. However, they sent me a sample of their cold-relief formula, and my cat got free of a serious bronchial problem after taking it for several weeks. (Yes, pets, children, and even plants have all been found to flourish on flower remedies. FES has an excellent monograph on using them with children.)

Flower Power in the Nineties

As we move into the Nineties, a great variety of new essences are being developed. New companies are coming into their own, and some of the major companies are joining together to address common concerns.

Delightful and potent remedies are being collected in the desert of the American Southwest, on the heaths of Scotland, and even in Russia. There are preparations made from seashells and elemental essences that tap into the Aurora Borealis. While information about the newer collections is not as well documented as Bach's, the process of making and researching the remedies is much the same, and the remedies are no less valid. In time, as the companies and practitioners amass thousands of case studies, we will understand them as thoroughly as we now understand Bach's. Perhaps you will choose to be part of this exciting discovery process.

In Appendices A and B you'll find more information about flower remedy sources.

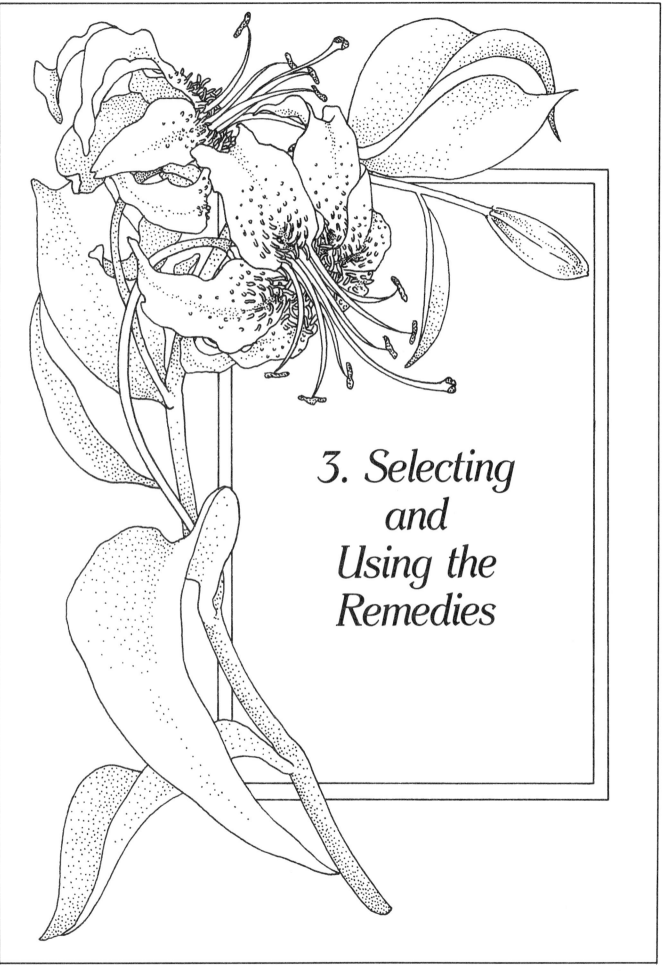

3. Selecting and Using the Remedies

OUACHITA TECHNICAL COLLEGE

Now that you've been introduced to the remedies, you'll undoubtedly be wondering which ones are right for you and the people you care about. In this chapter, you'll learn how to select them, how many to use, and the importance of checking the combination. You'll find out how to mix and take the essences and what to expect in working with them. We will also discuss some kinds of people who would be better off not taking remedies on their own. The instructions that follow will give you some guidelines, but listen to your instincts in using these essences, just as you would with other therapeutic methods.

How to Select the Remedies

Bear in mind that it's difficult to be objective in choosing remedies for yourself or a loved one. We can't always perceive ourselves or those close to us realistically. When our emotions are involved, we may see through rose-colored glasses—or, we may look at things in the most negative way possible. Being too close to the forest, we may not see the trees—or the flowers, for that matter.

So, where circumstances are emotionally charged—or the matters involved are serious—it's often best to consult an experienced flower essence practitioner. Almost all the essence companies offer consultations by mail.

ESSENCE DESCRIPTIONS

If you are working mainly for self-improvement, however, and feel able to be objective, there are a variety of ways to select remedies. Begin by reading essence descriptions in this book and in company catalogs or other literature. Thirty key remedies from a variety of companies will be profiled in detail here, beginning with the next chapter. For the Bach remedies, one of the best sources is Dr. Philip M. Chancellor's *Handbook of the Bach Flower Remedies*, available at health food stores and New Age bookstores. The Flower Essence Society has published an invaluable reference, *The Flower Essence Repertory*. The repertory describes and cross-references their own remedies and Bach's. For excellent literature about remedies by other companies, check the Bibliography.

TUNING IN

Once you have a list of likely-sounding remedies, double-check your selections through meditation. Begin by getting quiet, breathing deeply for a while, and asking your Higher Self to tune in to the flower in question. Some people find pictures of the flowers important in attunement, and there are drawings of more than 30 of the flowers in this book. However, there are other ways to tune in.

When some people hold an essence bottle, it feels hot when the remedy is good for them and cold when it is not—or pulsing with energy when they need it and inert when they don't. Others get a bodily sensation of moving toward the bottle if it is right for them and pushing away if it is not. Or, you may be like Dr. Bach himself, who would hold a flower and be inundated with the feeling it was meant to alleviate. Observe your own responses and signals.

THE PENDULUM

For many practitioners, a pendulum is easier to use. A crystal on a chain, a ring on a string, or any other dangling object can give you a yes or no answer, once you establish rapport with it.

To do this, get quiet, which is probably easiest to do while alone. (Some pendulums, also, are shy when other people are around!) Ask the pendulum how it moves when it means yes and when it means no. Some move side to side horizontally for no, like shaking the head no, and perpendicular to the body for yes, like nodding the head yes. Others move in a clockwise circle for one and counterclockwise for the other.

Start with questions you already know answers to: Are my eyes blue, is today Wednesday, is my name Jasmine? When you get reliable answers, be more daring. Ask ones you don't know the answers to but soon will: Will it rain today, will there be any mail, will my friend call tonight? When you're accurate with unknowns, you're ready to ask about essence selections. As you continue to get more comfortable, the pendulum has degrees of response. It may swing wildly when it feels strongly about your choice.

Be aware that you can influence the pendulum subtly if you are too attached to a particular answer. This is why major life questions shouldn't be settled in this manner! When testing for remedies, if you feel yourself wanting a yes or no, pull back and ask that the truth come through. Tell the pendulum to give the correct answer whether you like it or not. Double-check by asking if it's telling you the truth about a given question. For some odd reason, it always seems to answer that question truthfully!

MUSCLE TESTING

Others get clearer responses through muscle reflex testing. For this, you need a partner. Extend the stronger arm out in front or to the side at shoulder height. Resist with all your might while your partner tries to push the arm down, to get a sense of the natural resistance. Put the arm down and think yourself into the state of mind you want to heal, say, resentment. When you are consumed with resentment, put the arm out, and have your partner try to put it down. Most likely, it will collapse under negative states of mind.

Again think yourself into that state of mind, but hold the appropriate remedy in the other hand, near the solar plexus. If the remedy is correct, the arm should be strong again. Muscle testing is a good way to distinguish among similar essences, such as the Bach's many choices to take for fear. The strongest muscle test would indicate the right one.

CHECKING OTHER FACTORS

Experiment until you find which method is most comfortable and accurate for you. The important thing is to find a reliable manner of cross-checking your choices. Even when the descriptions sound as though they were written specifically about you and your difficulty, subtle factors may enter into the selection. Timing is perhaps the most crucial element. The essence must be appropriate to where you are right now in your healing process. Or, there may be a health reason why one is preferable to another at a given time. Without a double check, you may miss such delicate and often unconscious considerations. (The clearest check of all, of course, is to take your selections to an experienced practitioner.)

THE PAPER TEST

If you don't own a remedy and are wondering whether to buy it, write its name on a slip of paper and test that. If this sounds odd, write on slips of paper things known to be good for you—like exercise—and others known to be harmful—like arsenic. Fold them so the words can't be seen, and mix thoroughly. Test each slip in turn, then see what was written inside. If there isn't a strong negative reaction to arsenic, then the paper test is probably not accurate for you.

How Many Is Too Many?

When we first discover flower essences, the tendency is to want to take them all, because we identify with so many of the descriptions. In the Bach kit, for instance, many remedies deal with depression and discouragement. Having suffered with depression for many years, when I got the kit I decided to end this problem forever. I took all those preparations at once. The result was a horrendously painful catharsis—red, puffy eyes for days! Do yourself a favor and avoid this "kill or cure" approach!

How many is too many? Some teachers in the field say no more than four remedies should *ever* be given together. Apparently, Dr. Bach himself recommended no more than five at once. While this can be a useful rule of thumb, I have found in practice that some individuals at some points in time can handle no more than one. Others can assimilate up to eight of the exactly correct choices at the precisely correct point in time.

The Rule of Four seems to have derived from Michael Weisglas' important research project (discussed earlier). The group that received four essences showed the highest rate of improvement on psychological tests after six weeks. The group that was given seven remedies experienced more difficulty and tended to drop out of the study. Weisglas' tentative conclusion was that four was better than seven.

Although this information is persuasive, let's consider two points that aren't obvious in reading the study. One is that the remedies were not individually selected by experienced practitioners, but instead each participant received the same four or seven essences. It's true that almost everyone could benefit from certain remedies, such as the ones for guilt or for creativity, but timing is important.

Second, who is to say that some of the remedies were not operating at cross-purposes to the others? It's possible for essences to work at cross-purposes even when there are only two! To avoid this difficulty, test each likely choice. Then check the final selections for compatibility by holding a hand over the group of bottles while testing. If the response to the combination is no, keep discarding and rechecking until you find a group that works well together.

Matt Wood, a master practitioner and author of *Seven Herbs: Plants as Teachers*, says that odd numbers, like one, three, or five, are stronger and more dynamic than even numbers. In particular, he finds that his clients need either one or five remedies, seldom three.[1] Since Matt passed this along, I have been using odd numbers in combinations whenever possible, and they seem to produce powerful results.

More is not always more. There are practitioners like Matt who sometimes use only one selection at a time. They get excellent results by determining the precise remedy for the personality type. This is called the *constitutional* type or remedy. Over the years, the constitutional type for each of the 38 Bach Remedies has been spelled out. The best-drawn pictures of them are in Philip Chancellor's *Handbook of the Bach Flower Remedies*. For the more modern remedies, constitutional types have not generally been determined. The major exceptions are the richly detailed portraits given in Matt's *Seven Herbs*. They include Black Cohosh, Cat's-Ears (also known as Star Tulip), Easter Lily, Iris, Lady's Slipper, Sagebrush, and Yerba Santa.

Lack of in-depth knowledge often leads inexperienced people to overprescribe, shotgun fashion. In this addictive society, many believe that if two remedies are good, ten are better. Another possible cause of overprescribing is that the beginner may have a limited number of choices and only be able to approximate the correct one. After acquiring close to a hundred new essences in a recent year, I found that my precision was greatly improved.

What do you do if there are just too many excellent choices and the pendulum is enthusiastic about all of them? It's tough, but you simply have to set priorities. Choose those most relevant to the current concern, leaving long-standing but not acute issues until later. Also choose those that seem to enhance one another, so the mixture has a kind of theme to it. When two remedies are similar in nature, ask the pendulum if both are needed. Sometimes you can get along with just one of such a pair, but sometimes the two together are stronger than either is separately. Again, you wouldn't know this from reading the descriptions, but only from testing for that individual.

There are individual differences in sensitivities to remedies and the number of remedies indicated. In ongoing work with the same client, you'll find periods when he or she can take several remedies and periods when he or she can tolerate only one. During some periods, the client may need a break from taking any at all! Check the combination each time to determine the correct number.

For long-standing or complex problems, you may want to design a series of mixtures, as new layers and dimensions of the difficulty emerge. In ongoing work, there will be repeat selections and some new ones. When several remedies repeat—especially those that have been repeated more than once—they almost don't count in the total. Thus, ongoing clients are more likely to receive as many as seven or eight remedies.

Making Up the Mixture

Except with premixed formulas, like the combinations by Deva or Desert Alchemy, the bottles you buy are usually concentrates and shouldn't be taken in that form. (Bach's Rescue Remedy concentrate is an exception: it may be taken undiluted during a physical or emotional crisis.) The concentrates may be listed as *stock* bottles, while the diluted mixtures are known as *dosage* bottles. When in doubt, ask the supplier which type you are getting.

When you have made your selections, you need to mix the concentrates into a dosage bottle. A good container is the one-ounce (30 ml) amber dropper bottle that pharmacists use for nose drops or eye drops. Many pharmacies will sell you these bottles for about $1 each, or you may order them by the dozen from companies like FES or the Alaskan Flower Essence Project.

Sterilize the dosage bottle by boiling it for a few minutes and letting it cool on a towel. Put four drops of each concentrate you have chosen into the dosage bottle. Close the stopper and, holding the bottle by the top, pound it against your palm about 100 times, so that the concentrates are thoroughly mixed. Some practitioners recommend letting the mixture sit for a few hours after pounding so it blends together thoroughly. Some strengthen the blend further by putting it under a pyramid or near a crystal. Then, fill the dosage bottle nearly full of bottled or spring water. Again pound the mixture 100 times in order for the concentrates to permeate the water.

So that the solution does not go bad, it is best to add some form of preservative. Many people use a teaspoonful (5 ml) of brandy for this purpose. If you don't want to use alcohol, use apple cider vinegar. With a few exceptions, all concentrates you buy are preserved in brandy; the exceptions are Perelandra, Earthfriends, and, upon request, FES. In my experience, the few drops in a dosage bottle do not trigger drink signals for recovering alcoholics; but the especially wary could use the mixture in the bath instead of internally, or spray it around the room and over yourself with an atomizer. If, because of food sensitivities, neither brandy nor vinegar will work, keep the mixture in the refrigerator and watch for spoilage, which you will be able to taste.

Even if you aren't sensitive to alcohol or vinegar, putting several drops of the remedy mixture in your bath or in a spray bottle filled with water can increase the healing effect. These two uses enable the mixture to work directly on the energy field, clearing it out more rapidly. The bathing method is especially refreshing, in that you feel squeaky clean and deeply relaxed afterwards. The spray method entails spraying the rooms of your house—and even yourself—as a way to clear out accumulations of negative energy in your living space.

How to Take the Remedies

Generally, the correct dosage is four drops of the diluted version four times a day, or as close to that as possible. Taking the mixture more than four times a day does not get better results, except in crisis situations. To determine how many drops and how often, use the pendulum or muscle reflex test.

It's a good idea to take a dose in the morning, to get focused, and at night, to work with your dreams. Hold the drops under your tongue for 30 seconds for better absorption. If you used vinegar and don't like the taste, put the drops in water or juice. It is better not to put them into coffee or caffeinated tea, which may counteract the remedy's effects.

As you take the dose, think about the change you hope to achieve; or do related affirmations or visualizations. That "aims" the remedy through the power of intention. In taking a remedy for fear, for example, you might use an affirmation like "I HAVE THE STRENGTH AND CONFIDENCE TO COMPLETE THIS PROJECT." Several essence companies have composed affirmations for individual remedies, and others will be suggested throughout this book. However, the more specifically you design affirmations for your own situation, the more powerful the effect.

What to Expect

As you take the mixture, you may become more aware of thoughts and attitudes that create the unwanted pattern. That increased consciousness becomes the tool and the impetus for change. Dreamwork and meditation may be useful problem-solving tools now. As you become more and more aware of erroneous thought patterns, you may begin to find them uncomfortable and, ultimately, ridiculous.

For some people, the issue may actually feel a little worse in the beginning, because they're finally paying attention to it. It's like a nail in your shoe. You ignore it because you can't afford a new pair, but the day comes when you must get new footwear at all costs. All of a sudden the nail, which you've been tolerating by numbing that part of your consciousness, is unbearably painful. Consider it motivation, if you will. For others, the process is far more subtle. After taking the remedies for a few weeks, they become bored with their problem. They decide they no longer want to create drama that way, so they give it up.

If you lose interest in the mixture, forgetting to take it after a few weeks, it may have done its work, and it may be time to select a new one to address current concerns. Typically, you may want to repeat several remedies from the original mix, and add some new ones.

Be sure to test all the old remedies, so the work of that group will be carried to completion.

At times, however, new concerns emerge with such urgency that you have to pay immediate attention. The original selections may come up again later. Sometimes that happens because we regress under stress and go back to undesirable patterns; or we may grow in consciousness and need to approach the old problem on a deeper level.

As people work with the essences, layer after layer emerges—just as with other healing methods. For instance, in working with anxiety from unknown causes through Bach's Aspen, the underlying causes of the anxiety may rise into your consciousness. You would then want a new mixture to tackle those issues. If you're taking essences for aggressiveness, you may discover that was actually a cover-up for insecurity, so a new set of remedies is needed to develop confidence. If you were taking a remedy to release guilt at not having done more for a loved one who died—say Pine or Red Chestnut—you might find you were using guilt as a way of avoiding grief. As the grief surfaces, you'd select some of the excellent preparations for that, like Sturt Desert Pea and Bleeding Heart. Healing through the remedies is an ongoing process.

The Healing Crisis

The first few days you take a mixture, you may experience a catharsis of stored-up feelings or an apparent flare-up of symptoms. This is called a healing crisis. Not all people go through this stage, particularly if they've already done a lot of work on the issue. However, the first remedy a person ever takes may be the most cathartic, as the inner self rushes to let go of emotions that have built up.

This initial reaction is not unique to flower remedies. It's common with any form of healing, up to and including traditional psychotherapy. It's like what happens when you start a physical fitness program. For the first week or so, your body feels anything but better! You are pushing accumulated toxins out of your muscles and organs. And yet, as you continue to exercise, the results are worthwhile.

Some practitioners tell me they hardly ever find the "catharsis" response among their clients. Among mine, it is so common I was convinced such reactions were universal. Finally, it became clear that it has a great deal to do with the nature of the clientele—and the nature of the practitioner! A great many of my clients are recovering from addictions, adult children of alcoholics, abuse victims—or all three. Their life experiences are very difficult, and they stuffed many strong emotions in order to make it through. Other practitioners may specialize in young mothers, college-bound youngsters, or some other group that is generally functioning well but is under current stress. In this area, there is less chance of a backlog of unexpressed emotion.

Likewise, the practitioner's background may make a difference. One who is trained to be comfortable with catharsis and is experienced in dealing with it may "give a client permission" to release deeper feelings. A practitioner overinvested in drama may even tend to evoke it. One who is not comfortable with catharsis is likely to give out the message that such reactions are not welcome, thereby prolonging the healing process. Self-awareness and healing of the practitioner's own issues is the key to balance in dealing with clients' reactions.

Some practitioners advise against mentioning the healing crisis, believing that you create it by talking about it. I truly do not believe you can evoke a catharsis of emotions that are not present at some level of the client's psyche, wanting and needing to be released. It is more likely that by discussing the phenomenon of the healing crisis, you prepare the client for the possibility and give the buried feelings permission to emerge. When you don't discuss it, there's a good chance your unprepared client will just stop taking the mixture when the discomfort begins.

Let's look at two examples. One of my clients, something of a workaholic, was exhausted from a long series of deadlines. I gave her Bach's Oak and Olive. A few days later, she called in a panic to say that rather than having more energy, she got so wiped out that she had to go to bed for a few days. After talking about it, she finally saw that bed was exactly where she needed to be! She allowed herself extra rest over the next week and began to feel a new strength. As she continued to take the mixture for the next several months, she got smarter about pacing herself and saying no to extra assignments. Her periodic collapses stopped.

Another client was tormented with guilt, even though she was a conscientious person and considerate of others. I selected Pine, by Bach, as her constitutional remedy. At first, her feelings of guilt seemed worse, to the point where she couldn't look anyone in the eye. After a few days, she recognized that she'd always felt this way, although she generally was able to block it out. She wasn't guilty about anything specific—she was guilt on the hoof! She had been walking around for years, looking for the slightest misdeed to fasten her preexisting guilt onto. Naturally, childhood patterns and conditioning, which she came to recognize, were responsible.

Ultimately, she began to understand the way she took responsibility for everything that went wrong around her, and feel the absurdity of it. Whereas previously she would have been immobilized with guilt, she reported that after treatment, when she'd done something she wasn't proud of she was able to make amends, learn from the experience, and let it go.

Flower essences don't *cause* effects like the first woman's wipeout or the second woman's irrational guilt, but they *can* bring issues to the surface. The end result is strong forward motion. When an essence is taken through to completion, you develop healthier ways of thinking and behaving.

Catharsis may be important in releasing the pattern. Cry if you need to. Let yourself be angry, even if it's about something that happened twenty years ago. You don't need to act on the feelings that come up, or take them out on yourself or others. Just observe them and sit with them—they will change in a day or so. They aren't necessarily related to today, although they may be triggered by something that just happened. It's also important to avoid overeating, drinking, or taking drugs or pills to stuff the feelings back down.

If you are one of those people who reacts intensely, you may want to begin slowly. Take the mixture only once or twice a day until it feels comfortable to increase it. If more feelings come up than you believe you can handle, put the mixture aside and take Bach's Rescue Remedy, available in many health food stores, Desert Alchemy's Emergency Formula, or Aloe Vera, made by several companies. Work all the more closely with your support systems; take baths with seven drops of the remedy mixture in the water, and generally be kind to yourself. The storm will pass, and you'll be healthier afterwards, ready to work on basic issues that get in the way of wholeness.

The question is not whether the essences bring up feelings, but how willing we are to become different. Human nature being what it is, we often refuse to change until it is too painful to stay the same. We often go for help when we are on the threshold of change—hoping against hope that it won't be necessary to do it. We hope we'll be given permission to stay the same. Essences don't create change—only catalyze it—but they do support the person who is ready and willing to grow.

How to Learn About the Flower Essences

Although this book is organized as a reference guide, you may be wondering how to go about making the knowledge of essences your own. A good way to begin is to buy a notebook or one of those lovely blank books to keep notes in. As you try out a remedy, write down the condition or feeling you wanted to change, what the remedy and its description were, and why you chose it. Over the next several weeks, write down your reactions and the shifts in attitudes that occur. If friends or family members are also taking remedies, keep similar notes or ask them to do so and

to share them. When you've finished that formula, do the same with the next mixture, and so on. The shifts and changes occurring over time are instructive. As you keep records, you'll begin to notice when and why one particular essence might be used, as opposed to another.

In the subtle realms where flower remedies operate, it can be valuable to get the perceptions, insights, and experiences of a variety of authors. It's interesting how differently a particular essence is described by the various companies who make it. For instance, Aloe Vera is made by Desert Alchemy and FES. Desert Alchemy's description of Aloe Vera is that it relieves impatience with the healing process and resistance to allowing buried emotions to come up, so that there is patience and trust in the process. It also helps you to be in touch with the underlying joy of the healing crisis. On the other hand, FES says it restores life force energy when you feel burned out.

Having used Aloe frequently with clients, I have no doubt that both descriptions are true. In this subtle realm, writing an essence description is akin to the three blind men who were asked to describe an elephant. One had ahold of the trunk, the second the tail, and the third the massive flank—and each was convinced he had the last word on the subject! Like elephants, the remedies and their effects are far greater than suspected by those of us who are groping around, trying to comprehend them.

Therefore, you may eventually wish to read other books on the subject and subscribe to the newsletters put out by various companies. Some of the companies also sponsor workshops, so you might want to be on their mailing lists. It is useful to keep notes about what various authors and the companies making the remedies have to say. A card file or computer files would keep this information organized. I keep a master list of essences, complete with descriptions, to page through when considering which is right for a situation. As it is computerized, it is a simple matter to add new remedies and new insights and then print out an updated version.

Another practice that can be useful in learning the remedies is to meditate on a different one each night. Light a candle and put one drop of a remedy in a glass of water, stirring it. Clearing your mind and sipping the water slowly, breathe deeply and gaze at the candle. You'll start to sense the effect of the remedy, the feelings and attitudes it is useful in changing. Ideas about its connections with other remedies may also come through.

In this way I learned many useful things about the essences and their properties. For instance, when meditating on Oak, which is a major remedy for fatigue, I felt as though my body suddenly became the solid, massive trunk of an oak tree.

As I worked through a series of such meditations, I allowed the day's remedy to be revealed intuitively at the beginning of the session. The result was that relationships and connections among various essences became evident. For instance, the Bach kit has three remedies for fatigue—Oak, Olive, and Hornbeam—and I was initially unclear about which was appropriate in a given situation. After meditating on each separately, I learned they existed in a spectrum that can be characterized as follows: Hornbeam can provide relief if it's been a long, hard month; Olive is appropriate when it's been a long, hard year; and Oak is for when it's been a long, hard life. Reading the literature will clarify other differences—for instance, Hornbeam is primarily for mental fatigue—but understandings gained from meditation often provide fresh insights and a more direct grasp of the remedy than you can get from reading.

If you don't want to buy that many essences, try looking at the flower itself or a picture of the flower. That is sometimes evocative, especially if you're visually inclined. The 30 remedies profiled in depth in this book all have drawings to meditate on. The Peterson Field Guide series, published by Houghton Mifflin Company, is a good pictorial reference. Dover Publications publishes many inexpensive books of floral pictures. Many of the drawings used here come from their copyright-free series.

Dover's offerings include a series of flower coloring books. Coloring in the pictures is another good way to know the flowers, just a many people have learned the tarot by coloring in the black and white decks available for this purpose.

Of course, there are also good books on flowers in the public library, in botanical garden libraries, or in the botany departments of colleges and universities. If you feel like splurging, the Flower Essence Society has exquisite color slides of the individual flowers their remedies are made from. For those who respond best to scents, perfumed oils, candles, or potpourris are available for some of the flowers.

Remember the plant angels we spoke about in chapter 1? If you find that idea appealing, your meditations may become even richer if you ask the angels who work with that particular plant to be present. The Alaskan Flower Essence Project highly recommends their Green Bells of Ireland for attunement to the flower essences and their devas. It also helps you open your awareness to the various levels of energy and intelligence existing in nature. Other all-green flowers are said to have a similar effect.

And, finally, another way to understand the meanings of different flower essences is to study flower lore and symbolism. It is very useful to learn a plant's history, the healing properties that have been attributed to it in the past, and legends or stories connected with it. Interestingly, even when the makers of an essence aren't aware of the lore connected with a particular flower, their intuition often leads them to similar conclusions.

For instance, the remedy Basil is said by FES to help resolve conflicts between sexuality and spirituality or morality. Superstitious people ages ago regarded basil as a telltale herb because they believed it died immediately if the wearer was not chaste.

Dogwood is an essence that FES recommends for gentleness and grace in relationships. In the language of flowers, dogwood meant "love undimin-ished by adversity," and it is said to symbolize beauty, faithfulness, and stability.

The nettle plant symbolizes cruelty; in the language of flowers, it means "You are spiteful." Harebell offers Nettle as a remedy for cold, angry states, and it is often the colder form of anger that leads to cruelty and spitefulness.

Vervain is the Bach remedy for those who are incensed by injustices. The ancient Romans believed vervain had the capacity to repel enemies and considered it sacred to Mars, the god of war. They would send messengers wearing a crown of vervain to ask for peace—or, conversely, to carry a challenge.

Sharing the Remedies with Others

Once you've taken a few remedies with good results, you may want to share them with your friends. The essences, though, aren't that easy to explain. Let me start by saying that it's a good idea to be selective about the people you discuss the remedies with. The ultra-straight business person or traditionalist may find the idea altogether weird. The spiritual seeker is generally more receptive (and, frankly, tends to get better results with these subtle substances).

You might begin by asking if your friend has heard of the Bach remedies, as they are the best known. Many people have heard of them or even taken them—in which case, ask about their experience and proceed from there. For the totally uninitiated, you may or may not go into detail, depending on their interest. You might say that the remedies are based on flowers and other plants, but in a very diluted form, and that they help people mobilize to change destructive patterns in their lives. Mention one or two that seem particularly relevant, and ask if your friend would like to try them.

It might also be good to practice explaining the remedies aloud to a friend or a tape recorder a few times first, because hesitancy can communicate itself to the listener, who might then question the usefulness of the remedies. For the doubting Thomas, talk about the Weisglas study, and suggest trying the essences with an open mind. It's also an excellent idea to give some form of printed instructions to people along with the remedies, so they'll know how to take them and what to expect. Go over the information with them, clarifying any questions. It helps to let them know which remedies were selected and what each one is good for. That will sharpen their powers of intention and observation. Printed on page 39 is an instruction sheet you're free to copy and use if you like, so long as the copyright notice appears on it.

When you give a remedy to someone outside your immediate family, it's important to leave the door open for them to get in touch with you about any difficult reactions. Remember the cathartic effects remedies can sometimes have. Make it a practice to let clients know in a matter-of-fact way that these reactions can occur, that catharsis is often part of the healing, and that it generally passes quickly. In any case, you would want to provide for some kind of follow-up, since more than one bottle is often needed.

This might be a good time for me to talk about confidentiality. Even when you're just starting a practice, there are times when very personal information comes up as you discuss remedies with people. You are being entrusted with this information; your friends and clients are entitled to complete confidentiality.

Start slowly. You may want to purchase only a few remedies that seem to meet the needs of your particular clientele, family, or group of friends. Write down the date, whom the remedy was given to, what their symptoms and concerns were at the time, why you chose that remedy, and (by keeping in touch) what effect it had. In the same way, record repeat essences and changes in the combinations. There is much to learn, and your curriculum begins with the first remedy.

Are There People Who Shouldn't Use the Remedies?

Like all new converts, new flower essence users want to share their wonderful discovery with everyone they love. Now you know exactly what to do for your daughter's shyness, your aunt's hypochondria, your mate's grumpiness, and your best friend's lingering depression. Too bad they don't see it that way!

In my own work, I recommend essences to only about one in three. Over the years, it has become clear that some people really don't do as well on the remedies as others. There are also certain types whose dosage bottles grow green things in the refrigerator because they won't follow up on taking the drops. Here are the seven main groups you might hesitate to give remedies to, especially in the beginning:

- *People with serious health problems* or whose health is delicately balanced because of a sensitive constitution. Remedies can indirectly help with physical ailments, but it would be better for these individuals to work with qualified health care practitioners.

- *People who primarily somatize their emotions.* Included here are those whose emotions and conflicts are persistently expressed through psychosomatic illness, because they don't know how to deal with them more directly. These are people whose bodies are doing for them what they will not do for themselves—like saying no. Such individuals can have flare-ups of physical concerns when remedies bring up feelings they find difficult to handle. A skilled practitioner, one with a medical and psychotherapeutic background, may still be able to use the remedies with them. The newcomer, however, would do well to pass this sort of person along to a professional.

- *People who have been through too much lately* and are extremely stressed out or fragile—for in-

stance, those in the midst of, or directly after, a serious life upheaval or health crisis. Here, supportive remedies like Rescue Remedy, Self-Heal, Aloe Vera, or African Violet can mend and release the current stress. Don't give heavy-duty cathartics, such as Holly, Willow, or Bleeding Heart, which initiate the healing of long-standing, difficult issues.

- *People who are heavily addicted or on powerful tranquilizers* may not respond well to the essences. The addicted person may drink or drug even more heavily to deaden the emotions that come up. After all, they are addicted, in part, so as to avoid feeling in the first place. Although this is not always the case, people on powerful tranquilizers or antidepressants may not respond, or may respond unpredictably. Leave them to the care of their physician. If they really want to take the remedies, suggest they see a holistic physician.

- *People who aren't ready to change.* Many people, when they begin to notice that the old way isn't working, dig in their heels and refuse to consider that there might be a better way to operate. Respect their views and hold off, though you might let them know what's available.

- *People who are in love with their problems.* For these folks a chronic problem becomes The Beloved Affliction. The benefits of having the problem outweigh the rewards of getting well. They may get attention and nurturing they wouldn't get otherwise. Or, they may find it makes them important or enables them to manipulate and control others. You'll recognize them by the glow they get when they tell you all about Their Problem or their self-satisfied smirk when they explain why all your suggestions just won't work for them. (Bach's Chicory is tailor-made for people who use illness to get attention, but they may not be willing to take it.)

FLOWER REMEDY INSTRUCTIONS

NAME _____

PLEASE NOTE: No medicinal or psychotropic properties are claimed for these natural substances. You retain complete responsibility for following up on any necessary health care or psychotherapy.

You have been given the following flower or gem essences:

1) _____

2) _____

3) _____

4) _____

5) _____

6) _____

7) _____

HOW TO TAKE THEM: Four drops four times a day. In the morning, to get focused; at night, to work with your dreams. Hold under your tongue for a few seconds. Vinegar is used as a preservative. If you don't like the taste, put the dosage in water or juice. Cleanse the aura by taking a bath with seven drops. Do affirmations related to the desired change as you take the remedy.

POSSIBLE AFFIRMATIONS:

WHAT TO EXPECT: For the first few days, some people experience a catharsis of stored-up feelings or an apparent worsening of symptoms, in what is called a "healing crisis." This is an important stage in releasing the pattern. Don't act out on feelings that come up. They aren't necessarily related to today, although they may be triggered by it.

Important: Avoid overeating, drinking, or taking drugs to stuff the feelings back down.

As the healing crisis passes, you become more aware of thoughts and attitudes that create this pattern or attract this kind of situation. As you become more and more conscious of them, you begin to find them uncomfortable and, ultimately, ridiculous. This increased consciousness becomes the tool and the impetus for change. Dreamwork may be a useful problem-solving tool now.

For long-standing patterns, you may need a second or third bottle. If you lose interest in the mixture, it may have done its work.

TO REORDER: Return for a refill, or for a change in formula as new needs arise.

(Reproduced from the *Flower Remedies Handbook* © 1992 by Donna Cunningham, with permission of Sterling Publishing Co., Inc., New York, N.Y. 10016.)

- *People who aren't asking for help*. Sometimes a client asks for a mixture for a troubled lover, family member, or friend. Such people are not asking for help for themselves. They may be intending to give the essences to others secretly in their coffee or food. This is invasive, and constitutes spiritual malpractice.

So, yes, there are some kinds of people who may not respond well to the essences, at least not without expert guidance.

Where Do the Remedies Fit In with Other Methods?

If your continuing goal is self-improvement, no doubt flower essences are just one of the methods you're using to bring about personal change and growth. You may wonder whether the remedies will substitute for some of them, or how they would work along with the ones you've found particularly helpful. In chapter 4, we'll address these questions.

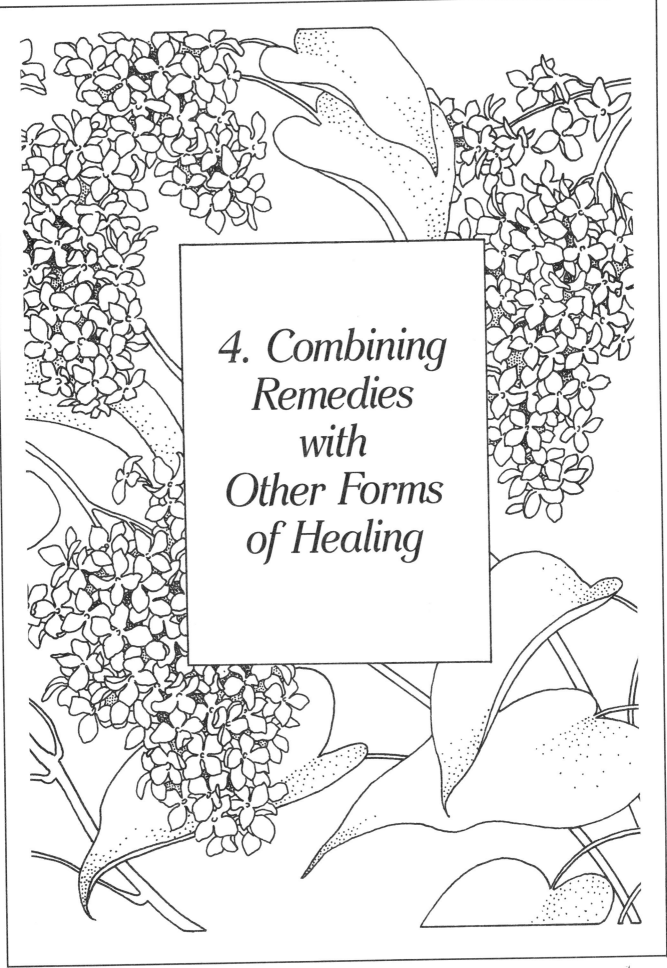

4. Combining Remedies with Other Forms of Healing

In this section, you'll learn how essences work with your chosen treatment methods to speed the process. Remedies complement traditional psychotherapy, group participation, recovery programs, bodywork, energy balancing, past-life regression, and a variety of other methods.

In later chapters, we'll discuss specific difficulties like poor self-esteem and painful relationships, along with relevant essences and such tools as affirmations and crystals that will further strengthen the effects of the remedies and make even more profound changes.

Some General Considerations

This book is an overview of the possibilities of flower essences. I will discuss most remedies only briefly, although we'll come back to important ones several times. In each remaining chapter, five key essences will be profiled in detail. Several possible remedies may be suggested for any particular problem. (Test to see which one applies.)

In order to make your selections, no doubt you will want more detail about their meanings and effects. This information is available from catalogs, brochures, newsletters, and casebooks provided by companies that make the remedies and from the books listed in the chapter notes and bibliography. *The Flower Essence Repertory*, for example, is an excellent source of information about both the FES and Bach remedies.

Many essences are made by more than one company. In the Appendix you will find all the remedies discussed in this book, and the names of companies who supply each one. In the body of the book, I mention the company whose product I use. Each of these organizations is reputable; none is recommended over another. I have merely credited the efforts of the company named in exploring that remedy and given the source of the description. Wherever possible, I have quoted the exact description given by the maker, because many of these are intuitively derived and each word or phrase may have some meaning that is not immediately apparent.

Remedies Used in the Healing Process

While there are many kinds of treatment, similarities exist in the attitudes that clients and practitioners bring to the process. Some mind-sets help—like self-acceptance and faith in growth process. Others hinder—like negativity, spitefulness, and fear of change. Let's begin with remedies that assist in healing, regardless of the type.

Self-Heal is made from the herb of the same name and traditionally used on wounds. True to its name, the flower remedy enhances people's abilities to heal themselves and to trust in the process. Taking it brings out inner resources that promote health and increase self-acceptance. It is paradoxical (*but sure*) that when we accept ourselves as we are, rather than condemning ourselves, we are more ready to give up self-limiting patterns. Made by FES, Self-Heal also comes in the form of a cream and a massage oil that can be used to speed physical recovery.

Remember that we discussed Aloe Vera in the last chapter. Desert Alchemy's description of Aloe Vera is that it relieves impatience with the healing process and resistance to allowing buried emotions to come up, so that there is trust in the process. It also helps people to get in touch with the underlying joy of the healing crisis. (In-depth profiles of Self-Heal and Aloe Vera, with their pictures, appear at the end of this chapter.)

Many practitioners describe Holly, by Bach, as an extremely important essence. Holly stimulates the release of deep-seated and unexpressed feelings, such as hatred toward others and the self and desire for revenge. With underlying attitudes like these, you may be dealing with someone who won't get well for spite. If these individuals believe that by giving up self-destructive patterns, authority figures, past or present, will "win," then they will probably find it very difficult to change.

The need for Holly is not always obvious, since most of us have been taught to hide unacceptable feelings and be "nice." So, test for Holly in the beginning, when you're dealing with persistent problems. Also, go back and test for it later if progress stops. (Holly is also profiled at the end of this chapter.)

Dealing with Discouragement

People with a chronic problem often seek assistance in many places. They may have followed a variety of regimens, submitted to a series of stressful and expensive treatments, and seen little improvement. Several Bach remedies are useful in such situations.

Gorse will encourage the individual to release that despair of ever getting better and help him or her to start again with renewed courage.

Crab Apple is a godsend for those who feel shame or self-disgust because of their illness or problem.

Impatiens will help those who lack patience in the healing process, getting frustrated when it doesn't move as quickly as they want.

Oak eases the sense of a long, hard struggle.

Where there has been a setback in healing, test for Gentian.

Kapok Bush, by the Australian Bush Flower Essences, is supportive for people who give up easily because of discouragement.

Borage, by FES, gives the person a quality of cheerful courage in facing up to challenges.

Dealing with Negativity

While sometimes born of discouragement, negativity is more often a learned pattern, perhaps soaked up in childhood. Muscle reflex tests show that pessimism seriously weakens us. Put your arm out, solid and strong, and think negative thoughts while your partner pushes down on your forearm. Generally, the arm will collapse. Most essence companies feature remedies against negativity.

Perelandra offers Okra, which they describe as especially useful for the gloom and doom type who sees everything in the worst possible light.

Among the preparations offered by the Australian Bush Flower Essences, Bauhinia is useful for those who are rigid and resist change.

Their Sunshine Wattle helps those who feel hopeless and expect the future to be grim.

Dealing with Hidden Agendas

We spoke earlier of people who unconsciously cling to a difficulty because it gets them attention and nurturing they wouldn't get otherwise. Some use emotional problems or physical illness to control family and friends, who wind up walking on eggs around them.

Bach's Chicory can help them release the need to gain attention in this way, so they can move wholeheartedly toward health.

To Aid the Client-Healer Relationship

Rapport and trust between client and practitioner are crucial.

FES's Fig, which is for trust issues, can be helpful here. Where the client's relationship with mother or father has been difficult, similar dynamics may come up in therapy.

The Flower Essence Repertory recommends Mariposa Lily where the mother-child bond was not good or was interrupted, and Saguaro for issues related to the father's authority.[1]

Desert Alchemy's Milky Nipple Cactus can also alleviate mother issues and excessive dependency that is transferred to the therapist or healer.

In the rare event that treatment becomes a power struggle, Vine, by Bach, may be helpful to both client and practitioner. Remember that practitioners can bring issues of their own into the session. Be sure to check out the remedies for codependency in chapter 8.

Remedies to Enhance Psychotherapy

The essences we are about to discuss would be supportive in any healing effort, but they are especially effective in psychotherapy. Some enhance insight into the deeper meanings and causes of troublesome symptoms.

Black-eyed Susan by FES is useful for clients who resist counseling and avoid looking at feelings. If you're ever going through a period of dragging your heels in therapy, try taking this remedy just before the session. It brings penetrating insight into emotions, as do Fig, Fuchsia, and Yerba Santa, made by several companies, and Scarlet Monkeyflower by FES. (A profile on Fuchsia appears at the end of this chapter, and Black-eyed Susan appears in chapter 6.)

Pendulum or muscle reflex testing will show which remedy to use—seldom is more than one indicated. The differences between them are not explained in detail in the literature. However, according to *The Flower Essence Repertory*, Fuchsia is more appropriate when repressed emotion comes out in psychosomatic ways and Scarlet Monkeyflower is especially recommended when the primary feeling being suppressed is anger.[2]

The FES catalog says that Yerba Santa ("holy herb") brings spiritual insight into emotions, particularly sadness. They also find it tones up essences that evoke painful or upsetting reactions.

Illyarrie, an Australian flower remedy made by Living Essences, helps us get by impasses that occur when we don't want to deal with something painful. Additional support for dealing with feelings will be provided in chapter 6.

A word of caution: Suppose an individual has used physical illness, addiction, compulsive behavior, overwork, fantasy, or some other distraction to suppress difficult emotions. When given remedies to bring feelings out, he or she will be all the more in need of therapy, healing, support groups, or friends who are willing to listen. Otherwise, even more strenuous efforts at repression could precipitate an increase in the symptoms. The person may also temporarily be more difficult to live with, as the real feelings, needs, and issues come out into the open.

Obviously, this particular group of essences is not to be administered indiscriminately! Don't give them to your husband or your best friend just because you think they are out of touch with their feelings and they won't go to therapy. Also do not give them without a clear explanation of what they are for and what to expect.

In particular, use the essences for dispelling illusions—like Bladderwort and Sand Dollar—with extreme caution and the deepest respect for the integrity of the individual. We cannot know what another person's life is really like. There are some whose illusions are the only things that make it possible to bear up under some secret hardship or sorrow.

For some people—but by no means all—an upsurge of symptoms may take place for a brief time, even with the best of support networks, as part of the healing crisis. Remember that any treatment, including traditional psychotherapy, can have this effect and is part of working the problem through. However, when you combine essences with such efforts, the clarity that results can be unsettling for a while. If something like this occurs, reread the section on the healing crisis in chapter 3.

Getting Unstuck

When an individual seems stuck in certain patterns or therapy seems to be going nowhere, several remedies help break a stalemate.

The Alaskan Flower Essence Project recommends Sticky Geranium for getting unstuck and going beyond previous stages of growth.

Cayenne is said by FES to catalyze quick change and overcome ingrained habits by mobilizing the will.

Bach's Chestnut Bud helps you learn from mistakes, so you don't keep repeating the same patterns.

Pacific Essences features Poison Hemlock for letting go and for moving through periods of transition. (If the name concerns you, remember that essences are vastly diluted, so no trace of any harmful substance is left.)

Regaining a Sense of Self

Near the end of the therapeutic process, there is a need to review what you've accomplished and get acquainted with "the new you."

You might try Golden Corydalis (Alaskan Flower Essence Project), which reintegrates the identity after a period of deep transformation, and also

provides a positive focus for growth of the personality.

FES's Sagebrush, which we'll be discussing in more depth in the chapter on self-esteem, is also useful in gaining a new sense of self after a deep change.

Working with Groups

There is great growth potential in groups, where the intentions of many join for a common purpose. A loving, positively motivated collective has more strength and power than any individual alone. Peers can encourage us to overcome blocks and move forward when we would be frightened to do so on our own. In particular, people recovering from the same kind of problem help one another in a way that outsiders cannot. We see this principle working in the twelve-step programs for

recovery from a large variety of addictions and compulsions, relationship problems, and dysfunctional family situations. Finally, while individual action does count, collective action is more effective in addressing concerns about the environment and other societal problems.

Yet, many of us hesitate to join a therapy, support, self-help, or social action group. We may fear their power or worry that we will lose our individuality.

It is true that groups can exert strong pressure to conform, but Goldenrod essence gives strength to retain individuality despite pressure. FES says that this is because it overcomes the tendency to present a false persona for social approval.

A further aid would be Trumpet Vine, which FES describes as supporting an active, dynamic projection of self in group or social situations.

Shyness and fear of not fitting in also keep many people from joining groups—or from participating fully. The remedies and healing tools for self-esteem in chapter 5 would ultimately make all social encounters less stressful.

Violet (FES) is the most specifically useful essence for being at ease in a group, since it helps you develop trust, openness, and warmth. It is especially supportive for those who experience shyness and fear a loss of identity.

Bach's Mimulus is useful for timidity; their Walnut is for strengthening those who are oversusceptible to the influence of others.

Chronic feelings of isolation and alienation make friendship and group membership difficult. They can be alleviated by Shooting Star and Mariposa Lily, made by various companies. (Shooting Star is profiled at the end of the chapter.)

FES's Oregon Grape relieves fear of emotional hostility from peers and encourages the suspicious or wary individual to develop trust in the good will of others.

Australian Bush Flower Essences offers Tall Yellow Top for alienation.

Where the person has had upsetting experiences in groups, either as a child or an adult, check out the remedies for trauma in chapter 7.

In social action groups and even some New Age situations, politics and jostling for leadership turn many people off and have often limited what a collective can achieve. A very special essence, Quaking Grass, could be taken by all members or especially those involved in decision making and political strife. FES says it blends individual egos and leads to group harmony for a common purpose, because negotiating skills improve. Undoubtedly, Quaking Grass would also be excellent for family conferences or family therapy.

FES also features Trillium for selflessness and putting aside personal desires for the common good.

Their Larkspur develops positive leadership qualities and charisma without self-aggrandizement.

Remedies for Recovery

As I mentioned earlier, many of my clients are in recovery from a variety of addictions, abuse, or dysfunctional family backgrounds. They have found the essences an extremely useful way of clearing out the toxic backlog of emotions that nearly always accumulates under such circumstances. Of course, remedies cannot replace the fellowship, guidance, and corrective life experiences that participation in recovery programs and twelve-step meetings provides, but as part of a holistic approach, the essences help people pass through the predictable crises of recovery. They

support the process of cleansing and releasing the accumulated fears, shame, resentment, and feelings of hopelessness and helplessness that make those first years of recovery so difficult. In addition, when people are no longer using substances to numb their feelings, they must relearn how to manage emotions sanely. The remedies greatly facilitate this process.

No one would claim that essences alone can cure addiction, but they do support the person who is wholeheartedly ready to stop and is pursuing other avenues of recovery as well. Some of these fall under the category of "hair of the dog that bit you" (the old homeopathic model of "like curing like").

An interesting experimental essence is *Cannabis indica*, based on the flowers of the marijuana plant. When its essence was given to several long-term pot smokers, some of them promptly disappeared, as active addicts often do. I suspect they simply didn't take the essence, because they were unwilling to change that particular pattern. However, two of the smokers experienced rather dramatic changes.

The first, who was not at all interested in quitting, took the remedy along with essence more related to his current concerns. When I spoke with him some time later and asked about his pot intake, he said that he hadn't been using it because he didn't have the money. Lack of funds, even for basic needs, had never deterred him from buying marijuana in the past! So, it did seem to me that the essence was in part a catalyst for the change.

The second man had struggled desperately to stop (with little success) for at least a year and a half. Much of that time, he was in therapy and attending twelve-step meetings off and on. Part of the difficulty was his relationship with an active alcoholic who would leave pot around the house. He was not in therapy at the time the essence was given to me for testing. He was told what it was and asked to report the result. Within a few weeks, he left town for the summer. This seemed like a positive step. Six months later, he had left the relationship, looked great, and was back in meetings. He had not smoked pot in that six-month period; he radiated calmness and strength. The remedy had apparently helped him turn a corner. Again, this is an experimental essence and much more research is required before it will be available.

In general, the person in recovery will find the remedies a source of support. Three considerations are in order, however: (1) Go gently and respect your instincts about when the remedies are right for you and when they are not. It is easy for the newly sober or clear person to overload, working compulsively at recovery with a variety of tools, and then to become overwhelmed. (2) Follow the instructions in chapter 3 about mixing remedies with vinegar, if alcohol has been a problem for you. (3) If you experience one of the healing crises described in chapter 3, follow the suggestions for dealing with it.

Remedies to Enhance Bodywork

Bodywork is an essential form of healing necessary to a holistic approach—and not just for those with health problems. Every disease operates on mental, emotional, spiritual, and physical levels, so true health comes about only when blockages on all these levels are cleared out. Many different disciplines are included in the bodywork category—from traditional medicine, nutrition, physical therapy, and massage to rebirthing, reflexology, rolfing, neo-Reichian therapy, acupuncture, acupressure, Jin Shin Jyutsu, and energy balancing. Earthfriends, described in Appendix B, offers oil-based essence and aromatherapy combinations for a variety of purposes that would be useful to bodyworkers.

The body has an incredible capacity to recall anything that has ever happened to it. Those who focus on a sore or inflamed body part and earnestly ask it to communicate are amazed at the layers of memories that surface. So, whenever there is physical trauma—anything from an accident to child abuse to rape—the body remembers and holds the shock until helped to release it. Psychotherapy can reveal why troublesome patterns such as fear of intimacy exist, but it's hard to change unless you also clear the imprint of the negative experiences out of the body.

Shock

Several remedies are useful in releasing shock, which can linger for years after the original incident. I have used bottle after bottle of Bach's Star of Bethlehem, since many clients suffered from abuse as children or from violence as adults. It is very potent in allowing the physical and energy bodies to let go of fearfulness. It is also useful after accidents or other sudden, terrifying experiences. Star of Bethlehem, profiled in chapter 7, is one ingredient in the famous Rescue Remedy.

The herb arnica is a well-known folk remedy for sprains, strains, and bruises. Many coaches haven't been at all embarrassed to use it for sports injuries. The flower essence Arnica speeds healing after an accident or injury. FES explains that it restores breaks in the life force after a shock. It reestablishes connection with one's Higher Self after severe physical trauma or injury. Arnica is available in flower remedy form, in essence-impregnated cream from FES, and in stronger preparations from homeopathic companies.

Many people keep an aloe vera plant around and break off a piece for cuts, burns, and abrasions, as its juice is very soothing. Aloe Vera remedy also enhances healing and restoration of life force energy after strain or trauma.

Releasing Fear from the Body

Numerous companies offer Dandelion as an aid in bodywork. It creates relaxation by releasing tension, fear, and repressed emotions held in muscles and organs. FES sells a massage oil containing Dandelion essence, suggesting the liquid remedy be taken internally at the same time.

For those who avoid bodywork because they are uncomfortable with physical contact or touching (especially males), Australian Bush Flower Essences offers Flannel Flower.

One of the goals of bodywork is better grounding in the physical realm, rather than living so much in the head. Various essences work on this need, including Madia, Manzanita, and Squash (all from FES).

Cleansing Essences

Two essences are known as cleansers on the physical level, as well as cleansers of the emotions. They are Crab Apple by Bach and Chaparral by FES.

Bach's Impatiens, for those who are irritable and impatient, can also relieve irritations and inflammations on the physical level. A friend was experiencing an eye irritation because of his contact lenses. We were at a conference center in the woods, with no doctor present. I suggested he bathe his eyes and lenses in water containing Impatiens. By the next morning, the redness was gone, and my friend had realized that he was actually very irritated about something that was going on in the group. This is a typical example of how the emotional and physical interrelate and how essences work on both levels simultaneously.

Remedies for Energy Balancing

Around and through the physical body are a series of subtle or ethereal bodies made of pure energy. These fields, also known as the aura, are visible to some psychically sensitive people. They include the *emotional body*, in which deeply felt emotions are either processed and released, or held and experienced again and again; the *mental body*, where ideas and thoughts are forever stirring; and the *causal body*, where strongly held beliefs magnetize experiences that tend to confirm these beliefs. The aura shifts constantly, in response to experiences and moods, but yet there can be frozen or stuck areas that keep the individual from growing or feeling free. Healing the causal body is rightly the territory of metaphysics, healing the mental body is a lifelong educational process, and healing the emotional body is the territory of psychotherapy.

Within the aura, there are centers called chakras. These are a bit like energy organs, corresponding to important functions. Significantly, they often appear in meditation and mystical drawings as flowers, so flower remedies have a natural affinity for them. The heart center is especially important, as it affects the ability to give and receive love. The solar plexus chakra (just above the waist) relates to self-esteem. The brow chakra (between the eyes) has to do with mental clarity, and the root chakra (at the base of the spine) with survival, security, and grounding. The crown chakra (at the top of the head) is the connection to our own soul and to the Divine.

We will discuss these centers in greater depth later. It is important to get a basic understanding of them here, though, because the aura may also need to be repaired before you can fully recover.

Negative experiences and dysfunctional family backgrounds may cause wounds or blockages, and it is hard to move out of the resulting patterns until the chakras are clear. We are drawn to or repelled by people mainly on an energy body level, even though many people have no idea it exists. When shock is stuck in the energy field, we tend to keep on attracting similar situations. When someone has worked hard to let go of toxic relationships, it is important to clear the energy field as well. Otherwise, such people may simply isolate in order to keep from repeating these painful patterns.

Several forms of healing focus on clearing out the aura. They include Reiki, MariEL, polarity therapy, Touch for Health, and the laying on of hands. Mentioned under bodywork, but operating at the borderline between the body and the aura, are Oriental arts such as acupuncture, acupressure, and Jin Shin Jyutsu, which align the flow of energy along the meridians.

In my observations of clients, the combination of flower essences and energy clearing is especially potent. Both operate on the vibrational level—more directly on the energy fields than on the physical. They work especially strongly when one is beginning a new remedy. There is a more profound release of unwanted patterns, with less discomfort.

We will learn later about remedies that alleviate wounds to various chakras. For instance, Fringed Violet, by the Australian Bush Flower Essences, treats damage to the aura where there has been trauma.

Earthfriends offers a set of oils, one for each chakra, that contain flower essences and aromatherapy products. These oils could be applied to the area of the body corresponding to the chakra when you are working on it. I use these oils regularly with my clients during sessions and in group meditations and find them very powerful.

Past Life Therapy and Regressions

Many practitioners find that persistent patterns and fears arise from damaging past life events, or even repeated events over the course of many lives. For instance, someone may have extreme fear of certain animals but never have had a frightening experience with them in this life. Others have repeated nightmares about fire, tidal waves, or catastrophes they have never experienced. Some relationships are inexplicable unless seen as karmic. In cases such as these, past life therapy can help the individual get free of disturbing patterns.

Some people who offer past life therapy or regressions are unprepared to handle the powerful emotions such undertakings can provoke. It is well to assess them carefully—and on a continuing basis—since no one can be accurate all the time. Dr. Roger Woolger, a Jungian therapist, has written an excellent book on the process: *Other Lives, Other Selves*.[3] For referral to qualified past life therapists, write to the Association for Past Life Research and Therapy, Box 20151, Riverside, CA 92516. It is a well-established and growing organization that holds conferences and training workshops and publishes a journal.

Several essences foster retrieving past life information and releasing associated emotions.

Petite Fleur's African Violet releases love and nurturing from the Higher Self, and thus would be strengthening during this work.

Comfrey, by Perelandra, is powerful in releasing and cleansing damage done by deeply held traumas, in this life and also from past lives.

Steve Johnson of the Alaskan Flower Remedy Project recommends their Soapberry for those who have a fear of nature because of some cataclysmic experience in a past life.[4]

Desert Alchemy has a series of formulas for those who seriously wish to pursue past life healing work: Unsealing the Akashic Records formula, followed by the Remembering and Releasing formula, and finishing off with the Ancestral Patterns formula.

Astrology as a Guide to Flower Essence Work

From the zodiac come the veritable secrets of God. The Star Angels are transmitters, and flowers become the symbols of their communication. The closer our communion with the angels, the deeper will be our sense of the mysteries of the plant kingdom and the greater our realization of the spiritual ministry of the world of flowers.

—Paracelsus

Connections have been made between plants and astrological conditions since earliest recorded times. Archaeologists have found ancient clay tablets in Sumeria showing that herbal work was done in conjunction with astrology. Physicians of medieval times and earlier considered astrology an important part of their studies. In fact, Hippocrates, whose oath graduating medical students still take, said that a doctor who did not use astrology should call himself a fool rather than a physician.

For medicinal purposes, plants were gathered under astrological conditions that, if not observed, were thought to make the medicines ineffective. The master herbalist Nicholas Culpeper who was born in 1616, recorded his conclusions about which herbs and plants correlated with the seven planets known at that time. Even now, herbalists and medical astrologers honor his designations.

There are also very strong connections between flower remedies and astrological conditions, which are listed for each remedy we profile. These connections hold true whether you are working with the birth chart, with ties between the chart and current planetary configurations (called transits) or with correct times to make or take remedies. I have used flower essences with astrology clients for ten years and find the combination superb. Astrology pinpoints the precise moment when people are most ready to release long-standing difficulty. The chart reading will show exactly when certain issues will be coming up for resolution. Dovetailing the right remedies for those issues with the right timing can produce a deep effect.

Astrologers might especially like working with the astrological combination formulas by Desert Alchemy. Made from cacti and other hardy desert plants, these formulas are very strong. One of the founders, Cynthia Kemp, is herself an astrologer, as well as a healer. There are formulas for transits from Jupiter on out, including Chiron. The Pluto formula, as you astrologers might imagine, really packs a wallop! There are also formulas for all twelve houses, so that having pinpointed one that is either loaded with difficult planets or else underdeveloped, you can use the formula for that house. For a brochure, write to:

Desert Alchemy
Box 44189
Tucson, AZ 85733

Another company that makes astrological formulas is Earthfriends, described in Appendix B. Theirs are oil-based, combined with aromatherapy scents, and are to be rubbed on the body.

Although you may not be an astrology student or know an astrologer who is also fluent in the remedies, you can use astrology in several ways. Through a chart reading with a professional, you can determine when particular issues become important and choose essences accordingly. If a professional reading is unavailable or too expensive, you might consider a computerized transit reading. Computers can't synthesize and individualize, but the newest generation of interpretations are written by highly regarded astrologers. The following are reputable services:

Astro Computing
 Services
Box 16430
San Diego, CA
 92116-9987

Heaven Knows!
1900 Peyton Ave.,
 Suite R
Burbank, CA 91504

Astrolabe
Box 28
Orleans, MA 02653

New York Astrology
 Center
545 Eighth Ave.,
 Tenth Floor
New York, NY
 10018

Daily, monthly, or yearly horoscopes in magazines or newspapers would not be an accurate guide to timing of remedies, as they are not personalized.

Whether or not you know your chart, there is still another way to make the remedies even more effective. The Flower Essence Society suggests that you begin taking a mixture at the New Moon and continue through the complete lunar cycle. One qualification is in order, however. Traditional astrologers believe that beginning an activity or project on the same day as the new Moon is unwise. However, by beginning it one day after, you make use of the long-known and considerable power of lunar cycles. The table shown below of New Moons for the next several years is adapted from my book *Moon Signs: Key to Your Inner Life*, which is intended to help the general public use the Moon's cycles.[5]

(If you or anyone you know regularly has a strong emotional reaction to the New Moon or Full Moon, I would recommend taking Queen of the Night, by Desert Alchemy, for several months.)

New Moon Dates—1992 to 1996

Here are the dates of the New Moons from 1992 through 1996. New Moons that are solar eclipses are marked E and indicate periods of stress, when remedy work can be especially helpful.

1992 Month/Day	1993 Month/Day	1994 Month/Day	1995 Month/Day	1996 Month/Day
1/4E	1/22	1/11	1/1	1/20
2/3	2/21	2/10	1/30	2/18
3/4	3/23	3/12	3/1	3/19
4/3	4/21	4/11	3/31	4/17E
5/2	5/21E	5/10E	4/29E	5/17
6/1	6/20	6/9	5/29	6/16
6/30E	7/19	7/8	6/28	7/15
7/29	8/17	8/7	7/27	8/14
8/28	9/16	9/5	8/26	9/12
9/26	10/15	10/5	9/24	10/12E
10/25	11/13E	11/3E	10/24E	11/11
11/24	12/13	12/2	11/22	12/10
12/24E			12/22	

About the In-Depth Profiles

In this chapter, we begin the detailed profiles of the 30 key remedies you have been hearing about. They include fascinating facts about a plant's history and lore, a picture of the plant to use for meditation, affirmations to use along with it, and the qualities of the essence itself. Additional information, such as the herbal or healing history of the plant and its unique growing habits or other properties, will also be presented so we can gain a better understanding of the remedy. In the appendix you'll find an explanation of the elements included in each profile and why they are useful to know.

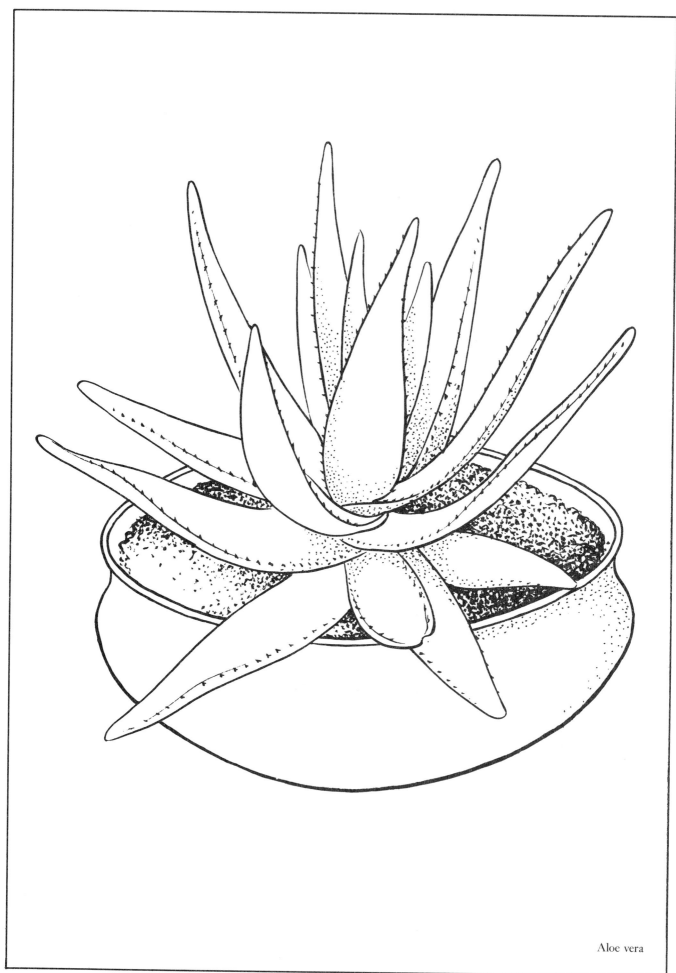

Aloe vera

ALOE VERA

Aliases: Latin name *Aloe vera*. *Aloe* was the native name and *vera* means a true aloe, as opposed to one of the variety of plants resembling it. Common names include burn plant and medicine plant.

Companies making the essence: Desert Alchemy, FES, Pegasus.

Essence qualities: FES's catalog says that Aloe Vera "restores life (etheric) energy when feeling 'burned out' or exhausted, especially from straining in creative work." Desert Alchemy's description of Aloe Vera is that it relieves impatience with the healing process, so that there is patience and trust.

Lore: In the Mideast, it had a strong association with Mohammed. Pilgrims would carry it to his shrine, then hang it over their home doorway on their return, for protection. It was also a funeral herb, planted on graves to give the departed a peaceful rest until the resurrection. Birthday flower for January 4.

What the plant is like: A cluster of thick, succulent blades arise from the center. The blades generally have prickly indentations, but are not sharp. Native to tropical and desert climates, it survives on little water and in very harsh conditions. However, it is grown widely as a houseplant, both for its healing and aesthetic qualities. The plant reaches 18″ to 20″ (45 to 50 cm) and has stalks of greenish-orange flowers that rise about 30″ (75 cm) from the center. They bloom every year.

Uses: Known for centuries as a healing herb, it was even mentioned in the Bible. The juice is soothing and mildly antibiotic, applied externally for cuts and burns, even sunburn. Internally, the powder is used for ulcers and as a laxative. Many people today grow an aloe plant on the window sill and break or cut off a piece as needed, squeezing the fresh juice onto a burn or abrasion. It is also used cosmetically for skin lotion and shampoo.

Reflections: This is a long-lived plant with many healing uses, and qualities of protection and resurrection are attributed to it. Therefore, it would stand to reason that the essence would have a restorative effect on the energy body and human spirit.

Affirmations: MY VITALITY IS FULLY RESTORED AND I AM WHOLE.

I HAVE ALL THE ENERGY I NEED.

I HAVE PATIENCE AND TRUST IN THE HEALING PROCESS.

Astrological correlations: To the Sun, which is the vital force or vitality of the individual. Thus, when having difficult transits to the Sun, such as from Saturn or Neptune, Aloe could restore energy and vitality.

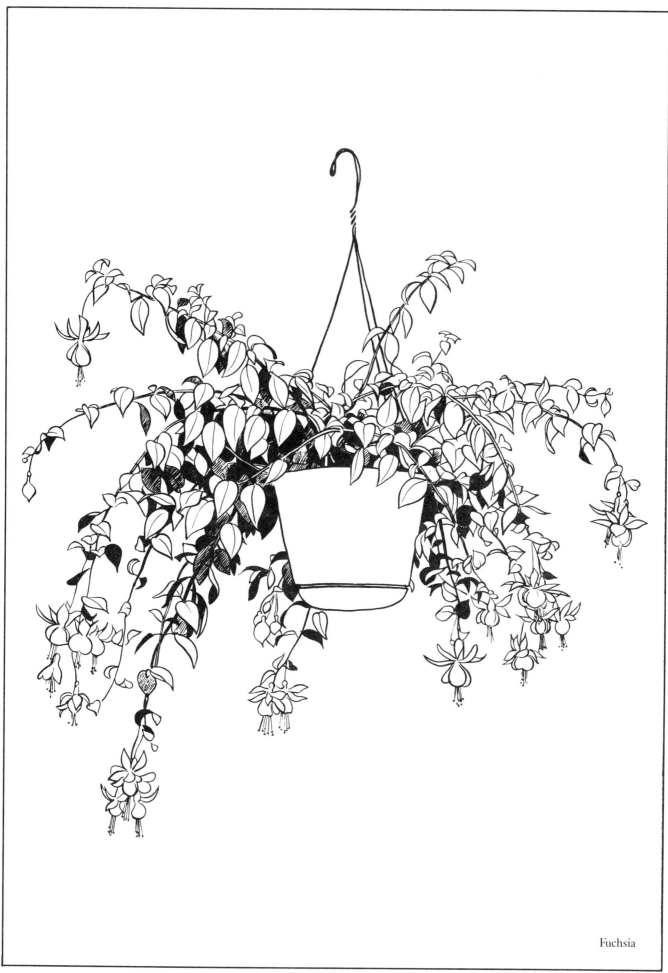

Fuchsia

FUCHSIA

Aliases: Latin name *Fuchsia hybrida*. Leonhard Fuchs was a German physician and herbalist of the 1500s; *hybrida* says the species used is a hybrid. One common name is ladies' eardrops, as the flowers are shaped like earrings.

Companies making the essence: FES, Harebell, Pacific Essences, Pegasus.

Essence qualities: The FES catalog describes it as facilitating greater awareness of repressed or deep-seated emotions like anger, sexuality, or grief, which are often expressed as hyperemotionality and psychosomatic illness. It can be a cathartic, leading to emotional release and greater emotional awareness. Helps those with psychological imbalances from early childhood.

Lore: Birthday flower for November 23. In the language of flowers, the scarlet ones carried the meaning of "good taste."

What the plant is like: Thick, bushy plants or shrubs with many smooth green leaves and richly flowering clusters of blossoms with their heads down. These shade-loving flowers are bright pink to red. The name of the color "fuchsia" derives from the pink ones. When kept moist the flowers grow nicely in hanging planters indoors, but not for long periods.

Uses: Decorative only.

Reflections: The *FES Journal* points out that fuchsia's heyday of popularity was Victorian England, when there was particular difficulty in dealing with anger and sexuality and much sublimation into such hysterical manifestations as fainting.[6] The language of flowers meaning of good taste no doubt stems from the Victorian disapproval of openly expressed emotion.

Affirmations: I PERMIT MYSELF TO KNOW MY DEEPEST FEELINGS.

I ACCEPT MY FEELINGS WITHOUT CONDITION.

I RELEASE MY EMOTIONS SAFELY BUT SURELY.

Astrological correlations: The Moon shows how people deal with emotions, and people with the Moon in Pisces or connected with the planet Neptune often need this remedy, as they tend to repress feelings. The Moon in Virgo may also follow this pattern.

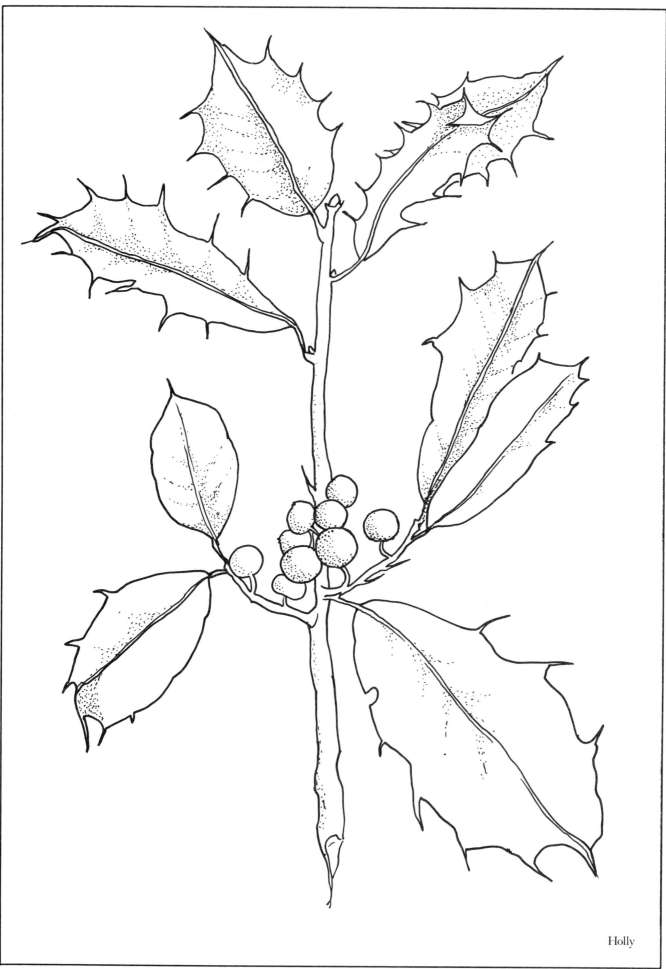

Holly

HOLLY

Aliases: Latin name *Ilex aquifolium*. *Ilex* was the common name used for a holly-like tree; *aquifolium* comes from *acus* (needle) and *folium* (leaf). Common names include holy tree, Christ's thorns, and bat's wings.

Companies making the essence: Bach, FES, Healing Herbs, Pegasus.

Essence qualities: This essence helps people let go of the most toxic emotions, including self-hate, hatred, jealousy, envy, suspicion, and the desire for revenge.

Lore: Roman emblem of goodwill, sent as a gift during the feast of Saturn, from the 17th to the 19th of December. Celts used it as decoration at the winter solstice, to defend against witchcraft and to protect the house from lightning. Holly water was sprinkled on newborns to protect them. Druid astrology sign for July 9th through August 5th. In the European flower calender, it was the flower of the month for December. Birthday flower for March 5. In the language of flowers, it meant "Am I forgotten?"

What the plant is like: A tree or shrub growing to 45′ (13.5 m) with hard, shiny, green scalloped leaves with needle-like tips. The tiny blossoms are white or pale green, with four to six petals and lightly scented. There are red berries, but only if you plant a male and a female plant together.

Uses: The leaves, berries, and bark were all used medicinally, for different purposes. Holly was used to cure fevers, as an astringent, and to induce vomiting, which was once an important element in standard medical practice. The berries were believed to help people who had gas and were used to alleviate colic and diarrhea. The bark was used against malaria. The juice of the leaves was used against tetanus. The plants would be tied around meat that was being preserved, to keep the rats away.

Reflections: So long as emotional habits like hatred, envy, or spite are present, the person is likely to avoid getting well out of spite. Said by many to be an important essence in "clearing the case," Holly is often given first or when the person seems to be at an impasse.

Affirmations: I RELEASE ALL THE HATE IN MY BEING.

I RELEASE THE HABITS OF JEALOUSY
AND ENVY.

I LET GO OF ALL SPITEFUL BEHAVIOR.

Astrological correlations: Often needed by people with Scorpio or the planet Pluto strong in their charts—for instance, when the Sun, Moon, or Ascendant is aspected by Pluto or is in Scorpio.

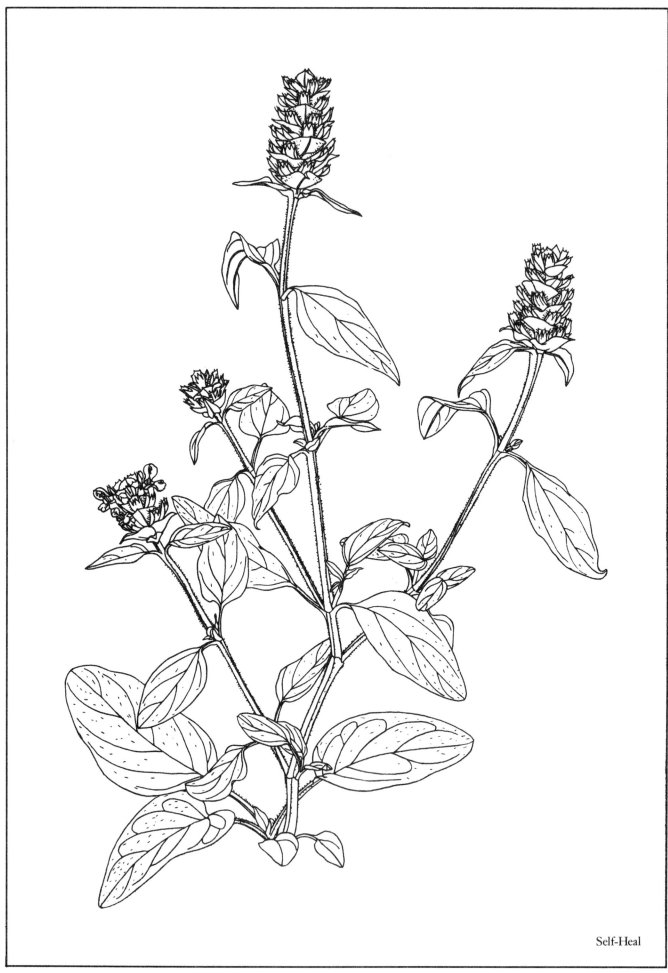

Self-Heal

SELF-HEAL

Aliases: Latin name *Prunella vulgaris*. *Prunella* comes from the German word for prune: *vulgaris* means common or garden variety. Common names include all-heal, carpenter's herb, heart of the earth, woundwort, and blue curls.

Companies making the essence: FES, Pegasus.

Essence qualities: FES says that it enhances self-healing powers and helps increase self-confidence and self-acceptance. It allows trust in the self-healing process, especially for those who have tried many healing modalities without success. It brings out inner resources for health.

Lore: As self-heal meant "that with which one may cure oneself without the help of a surgeon," it was widely said, "No one wants a surgeon who keeps self-heal." Because these flowers are shaped like a mouth, it was believed that the herb was good for mouth inflammations.

What the plant is like: This member of the mint family grows 1′ to 3′ (30 to 90 cm) high. The seed looks like a small ear of corn. It blooms from June to September, with spikes of dense yellow or purple flowers with two lips.

Uses: It was considered the best of all herbs, grown by a great many people as a home remedy. It was used against worms, as a mild diuretic, as a gargle for throat irritation, for kidney and bladder stones, and for toothache. Its common use by laborers for all cuts and wounds led to the name of carpenter's herb. Native Americans combined it with catnip for a laxative. They also made it into a tea that they drank to sharpen their powers of observation for hunting and tracking.

Reflections: Chiropractic is based on the belief of the innate wisdom of the body to heal itself. This essence might especially resonate to the chiropractic system of health care. This important adjunct to essence work might be tested early on in any course of treatment.

Affirmations: I TRUST IN MY ABILITY TO HEAL MYSELF.

I LISTEN TO AND HEED THE INNER CLUES TO HEALING.

I EMBRACE THE INNATE WISDOM OF MY BODY TO HEAL ITSELF.

I RELEASE ALL BELIEFS OF HELPLESSNESS.

Astrological correlations: Strengthens the vitality of the Sun, which is the center of the life force, but might also be taken with—or in anticipation of—any difficult transit by an outer planet (Saturn, Uranus, Neptune, or Pluto) to a planet in the birth chart.

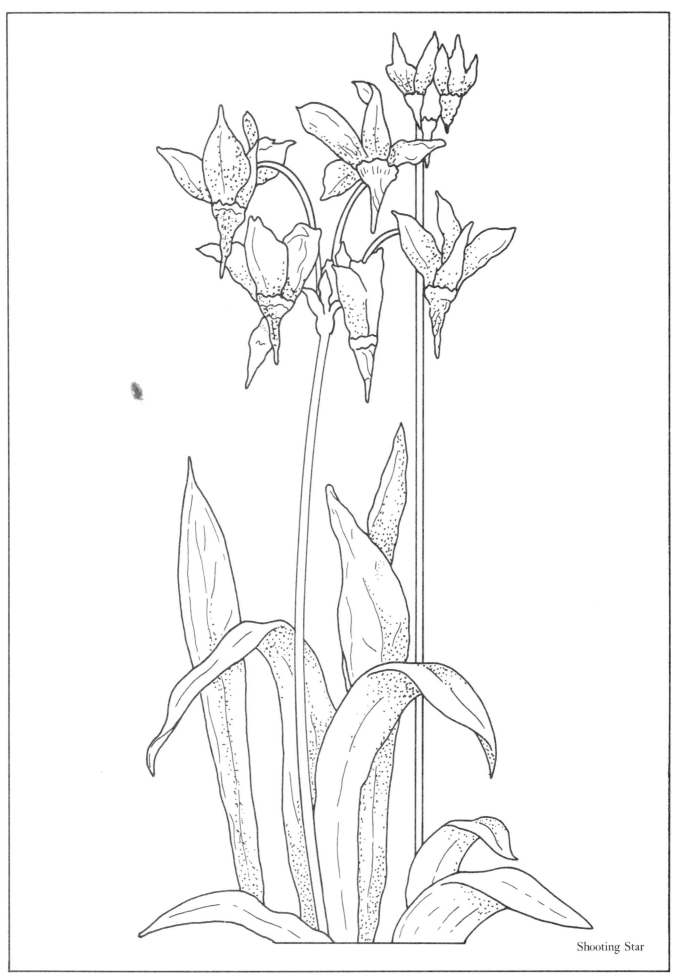

Shooting Star

SHOOTING STAR

Aliases: Latin name *Dodecatheon meadia*. *Meadia* after the botanical patron, Richard Mead. *Dodecatheon* comes from two Greek words: *dōdeka* (twelve) and *theos* (god). Thus, the name hints at a connection with the 12 zodiac signs. Common names were pink comet and prairie pointer.

Companies making the essence: Alaskan Flower Essence Project, FES, Pegasus.

Essence qualities: FES says it helps with feeling at home on earth and with others; also for overcoming profound soul alienation among those who feel they don't fit in.

Lore: In the language of flowers, it meant "You are my divinity."

What the plant is like: Blooming in late spring, the pink to crimson petals point skyward on an arched stem, with the yellow center pointed earthward, so that the blossoms resemble a starburst. These plants were once very common on the American prairies and in the West, but are now harder to find. The flowers are 1″ (2.5 cm) across and the stems are about 18″ (45 cm) tall. They are particular about their growing conditions. If it is not moist and rather cool, with good weather, they will either delay flowering or refuse to flower at all. They also respond poorly to being transplanted; they resent being disturbed. Although delicate in appearance, they are survivors, retreating underground when there has been a drought or fire and reseeding when conditions improve. Cyclamen is a tame relative.

Uses: One book called it a perennial herb and suggested there were medicinal uses, but subsequent research did not reveal any.

Reflections: Each quality of the plant resonates to the essence meaning. There is a joyfulness and exuberance in the brightly colored blossoms, the shape a clear indication of wisdom coming from heaven down to earth. The flowers grow in clusters, off the same stalk, a reminder that we are all related even though we take different paths.

Affirmations: THERE IS NO SEPARATION OR ALIENATION.
I BELONG TO HUMANITY AND IT TO ME.
I AM ONE WITH THE UNIVERSE.

Astrological correlations: Useful for "outer planet people," those who feel like aliens because of the predominance of Uranus, Neptune, and Pluto in their charts.

Moving On to Your Issues

We've looked at ways flower remedies can enhance your choice of treatments—everything from psychotherapy and bodywork to Reiki and astrology. Now, however, it's time to get moving on the issues that most often create blockages to happiness. We'll begin with one of the most common—low self-esteem—and it might be useful to begin your work there too. After all, low self-esteem is often at the bottom of difficulties in relationships, career, and even family conflicts.

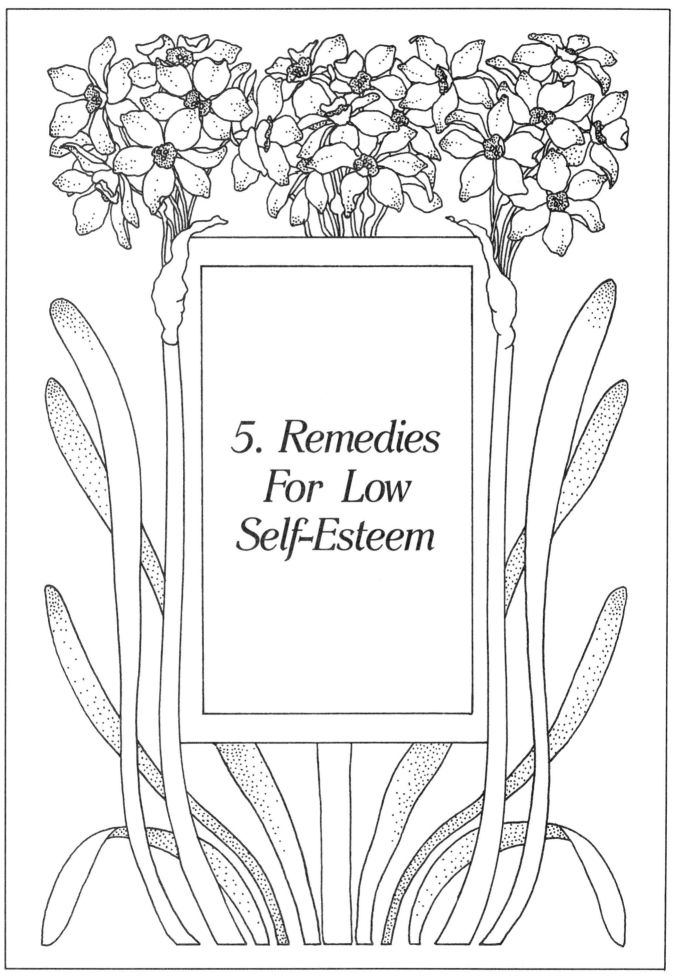

5. Remedies For Low Self-Esteem

Low self-esteem—how many times has it been a major stumbling block to happiness and success? How many times have others blithely told a self-hating person, "You have to love yourself first, before anyone else can." But how does a person go about doing that? This chapter will provide some suggestions.

One of the most frequently encountered of the modern ills, low self-esteem is nearly as frequent as the narcissism that is its underbelly. When a person has a poor self-image, you can rave about his talents, potentials, and good qualities, but he won't believe it. Worse, he may use his undeveloped potential as a reason for further self-hate.

Low self-esteem is also a major reason people get hooked into abusive and demeaning relationships. When people feel bad about themselves, they may either allow others to treat them badly or may treat others badly in order to feel better about themselves—or both.

Who Taught You That You Weren't Lovable?

When adults talk to children, the hurtful things they say are rather shocking. Shaming, blaming, destructive criticism, and character assassination are all too frequent in these exchanges, in the name of discipline. When done habitually, they contribute to low self-worth in adulthood.

To identify sources of self-hate, write down the most memorably painful things parents or other crucial adults like teachers said to you and about you. The messages absorbed may still be present in the mean things you say to yourself. Work to offset the power of such statements by writing CANCEL over them and tearing them up, flushing them away, or burning them.

Sometimes parents are supportive, but children learn to feel unacceptable because they are different from those around them. As a therapist, I often find that ridicule or harsh criticism by teachers has damaged children's confidence in their abilities. Peers, too, can be cruel, and the memory of not fitting in as a child can make the adult feel inadequate in social situations.

Unhappy childhood memories can be eased with Golden Eardrops, by FES. This remedy can initially have a cathartic effect, so if it does, use the hints given earlier about the healing crisis.

Many therapists, healers, books, and workshops are available to work on healing the inner child. If you felt unloved or were hurt as a child, they can foster learning to love yourself. We will also learn about flower remedies and other tools to use in the quest to heal the unloved child within and to let go of rejection. Self-hate is especially common to adult children of alcoholics, victims of abuse, and others who grew up in dysfunctional families. Scars from family traumas or difficult childhood experiences outside the family cannot be healed by flower essences alone, but we will discuss some tools in chapter 7.

The Effects of the Media

Even where parents were loving and supportive, where school was positive, and where friendship was rewarding, there are still many ways for self-esteem to be damaged. We live in an era where the media set standards for acceptability, based on externals like appearance, wealth, and career accomplishments. We are under constant comparison to the beautiful people portrayed on television, in movies, and in advertisements. With continual exposure to physical perfection, success, and wealth, few can measure up. Even if we match up in one area, we may feel like losers when we cannot excel in all.

Women are expected to look perennially twenty, with the body, face, and wardrobe of a fashion model. Additionally, women are pressured to be brilliant in a career, have a lovely, always spotless home, cook gourmet meals, and be an enlightened parent. No one can juggle all these demands without stress. Yet, when they cannot, women think less of themselves.

Japanese Magnolia, by Petite Fleur, paves the way to reconciling these demands.

Men are under pressure as well, to progress in their careers, to remain youthful-looking and slim, and to score sexually. Relationships suffer from these comparisons too. The media condition us to look only for the perfect, fantasy lover, creating unrealistic desires and demands for the dream girl or guy.

For joyful confidence in the attractiveness of your essential self, FES recommends Wallflower.

For low self-esteem based on dislike of one's appearance or body, Australian Bush Essences recommends Five Corners.

Flower Essences for Self-Esteem

Certain remedies can have a significant positive impact on self-esteem; almost all my clients get them at some point. Some of the finest remedies for such problems come from FES.

Self-Heal, which has many uses, is good for restoring confidence.

Sunflower is a major one for the ego, whether there is too little or too much. It balances the self-esteem, so the person is neither self-hating nor arrogant, but instead has a strong sense of self-worth, along with a lovely humility.

Another sunny yellow flower, Buttercup, is listed in the FES catalog as helping you value your own gifts and appreciate your worth. Almost everyone could benefit from this very special essence, but it is especially good for people who do creative work or whose job involves constant pressure to perform. My New York City clients used up one stock bottle in just four months. Both Sunflower and Buttercup will be profiled in this chapter.

As an example of what Buttercup can do, I gave it to a young professional woman whose self-esteem was low. I added Gorse for despair and Holly for her resentments toward family members. She experienced a strong emotional catharsis and felt too uncomfortable to continue, so she stopped taking it after only two weeks. Five months later, she contacted me for a new remedy. She reported that following the short period of taking the first mixture, she had suddenly renewed an interest in singing and acting which she had abandoned seven years previously, and she was taking classes for them. I had not given her the mixture for that purpose, but such had been the serendipitous side effect. No other new circumstances had arisen to account for this change.

Shame also arises when we feel someone else has put us down, and for those occasions Living Essences of Australia suggests Dryandra. Often, a rejecting parent started the cycle of shame, and in those cases Dryandra may be required over a longer period of time. In the next chapter, we will look at the closely related emotion of guilt, which also contributes to self-hate.

Alexis Rotella has identified Indian pipe as a plant whose essence would be especially helpful for Native Americans in coming to terms with their oppression. However, she experienced difficulty in making the essence. As soon as this albino plant is picked, it begins to turn black! I see this as somewhat of a signature, symbolizing the days of darkness that began for Native Americans when they were removed from their natural environment. Alexis feels Indian Pipe would also be useful for those who are studying Native American shamanism. (Pegasus now offers this essence.)

True self-esteem comes from accepting and expressing who we are, rather than being ashamed and hiding it. Goldenrod, by FES, helps us to remain true to our individuality rather than present a false persona for social approval.

Their Mullein, which is profiled later, helps us be true to ourselves and fulfill our real potential.

Sometimes, even as adults, we are different and don't get much validation. The Australian company Living Essences advises Yellow Cone Flower when we feel a lack of recognition from others. It fosters letting go of that need and realizing that the important thing is how we feel about ourselves.

Bailey Essences from Great Britain suggests Bracken for frustration and dejection from a chronic inability to express one's true self in the world. It is especially intended for the person who continues to play a child role in adult life.

We don't always have a clear picture of who we are. Our sense of self needs to change as we do, but we often outgrow it as we progress. The Alaskan Flower Essence Project features two remedies that help us let go of outdated self-concepts. The catalog describes Yellow Dryas as allowing individuality to unfold, providing expansion and clarification of one's true identity throughout cycles of growth and change.

Their Golden Corydalis is said to promote reintegration of one's identity after an experience of deep transformation.

FES's Sagebrush is an important remedy for letting go of false self-images that no longer serve a productive purpose. (Sagebrush is profiled at the end of this chapter.)

A Combination for Identity

In my ongoing work with clients, I find that many allow themselves to be limited through identification with their families. The combination of Sagebrush and Sunflower from FES and Honeysuckle by Bach is a powerful formula for releasing such patterns of identification. (Honeysuckle is a remedy for nostalgia and for letting go of the past.) As you experience these essences, you gain new insights about how you have held yourself back by internalizing family limitations.

The combination is particularly useful for the upwardly mobile who have come from poverty and hardship. They are frequently conflicted about surpassing their parents and threatened by losing their roots. This conflict sometimes leads them to self-sabotage. It is painful to go beyond one's roots when there are no models, particularly when parents never had an education or buried their own talents and dreams because of family responsibilities. Such upwardly mobile individuals are often simultaneously encouraged and covertly threatened with abandonment by less fortunate or able family members, who are envious or disparaging. Oak might also be added to ease the long, hard struggle they have had.

For example, one client of mine had come a long way from his origins in a very poor family. No one in his family, for several generations, had so much as graduated from high school. Yet, with scholarships, he had managed to complete a master's degree. As the years went on, he always managed to be on the brink of financial disaster, just as his siblings continued to be—even though his work was excellent and he had gained recognition in his field. I prescribed the Sunflower/Sagebrush/Honeysuckle combination twice, along with the affirmation I RELEASE MY ATTACHMENT TO MY FAMILY'S POVERTY. He realized he'd been staying broke out of a misplaced loyalty that neither helped his family nor brought him any closer to them. Within weeks, he landed a lucrative contract, which proved to be the basis of a much sounder life-style.

The same combination can be useful at the opposite end of the spectrum, when the individual has a very successful or celebrated parent—a wealthy father, for example, or a very beautiful and talented mother, whom the person is always compared to. This can be devastating to self-esteem, especially where there are remnants of the younger self who had no hope of measuring up, and where the parent was consciously or unconsciously competitive. (In order to be successful in the first place, the parent almost had to be competitive by nature.) Here the combination restores the person's confidence, so that he or she can find a unique path and identity.

In general, the Sunflower/Sagebrush/Honeysuckle combination helps loosen old definitions of the self. Perhaps it is a lingering self-image as a graceless teenager or a hick. Even though transformative experiences have brought a new way of being, the older concept may surface, causing self-doubt or self-hate. The combination helps to anchor to a new and expanded understanding of the self. Since all of us who work with essences are continually transforming ourselves, I would recommend a trial bottle of this mixture to almost anyone.

Affirmations to Create Self-Love

In several of her books, metaphysical healer Sondra Ray suggested writing the same statement 70 times a day for seven days.[1] She says that 70 times 7 is a magical number of completion. I have found this tool to be an exceptional catalyst. The mind has to be deprogrammed before it can be reprogrammed. A self-defeating or self-hating belief has been repeated over and over mentally for years, so it has to be confronted directly and undone—a redeciding. Otherwise, it counteracts positive affirmations—and then you wonder why they don't work!

This tool is especially powerful in working for self-worth. For example, you might write, "I RELEASE MY SELF-HATE," or "I RELEASE ALL UNREALISTIC EXPECTATIONS OF MYSELF." When used with a flower remedy or combination directed at improving self-esteem, this release work is especially catalytic. Many of the companies offer affirmations to go with their remedies. Anything you can do to personalize them and make them specific to your own situation increases their effectiveness.

Try out possible statements on a pendulum or muscle reflex test until you get the strongest combination. In particular, listen to the judge and jury inside to identify self-hating statements so you can deprogram them. Here are some affirmations to try:

I RELEASE MY PARENTS' OPINIONS OF ME. The word OPINION is useful here, as it covers both negative and idealized concepts. Your parents' judgments, beliefs, criticisms, disappointments in you, and prophecies of how you were going to turn out were all only that—opinion, not fact. Give some thought to what those opinions, beliefs, or judgments were. It may be productive to work on your mother and father separately. If other members of the family made troublesome judgments, choose the more inclusive word FAMILY'S rather than PARENTS'. Saguaro, by FES, helps you deal rationally with parental authority, and Dryandra eases the sense of rejection.

I RELEASE ALL UNREALISTIC EXPECTATIONS OF MYSELF. By ALL we understand not just your own, but your family's, lover's or mate's, friends', colleagues', and the culture's expectations. Cymbidium, by Harebell, makes it possible for us to be less frightened of others' disapproval.

I RELEASE MY IDENTIFICATION WITH MY FAMILY'S _____. In the blank, put any family pattern you may be carrying on despite its unsuitability or undesirability for you as an individual. For example, it might be their poverty, negativity, addictions, failures, unhappy marriages, or frustrated creativity. Sagebrush would be especially good to take along with this one.

I RELEASE ALL PAST EXPERIENCES OF FAILURE. ALL may denote past life experiences or even family members' failures that you soaked up psychically or felt reflected on you. Larch or Gentian by Bach would be strengthening. Alaska's River Beauty helps you start over again after a devastating experience.

I RELEASE ALL COMPARISONS OF MYSELF TO OTHERS. This includes the media, people in higher (or lower) positions, and those with more appeal, money, or accomplishments. Wallflower and Columbine would be useful.

I ACCEPT AND LOVE MYSELF AS I AM. This does not mean you won't continue to work for change, but it proclaims that you are loveworthy though imperfect. Dryandra or Correa may be indicated, as well as Beech.

I CHERISH MY INDIVIDUALITY, MY SPECIAL GIFTS, AND MY CREATIVITY. Philotheca, by Australian Bush Flower Essences, allows people to accept acknowledgment and speak of their success. Columbine, Alpine Azalea, or Mullein may also be helpful.

I AM RICHLY NOURISHED BY MY HIGHER SELF. For some, SOUL is a more meaningful word. African Violet is a remedy that would work especially well with this affirmation.

A word of explanation to students of metaphysics: You've undoubtedly heard that "affirmations should always be stated as positives." This time-honored rule basically applies to the words "no," "not," or "never." But syrupy affirmations like "Love and abundance flow into my life" very often don't work, no matter how earnestly you recite them. Strong underlying beliefs that contradict the positive affirmation can counteract all the hard work people put into them.

Core beliefs such as "I will never be loved" have been repeated inwardly thousands of times. A stubbornly entrenched belief system must be confronted head-on in order to change a long-standing pattern. You can deprogram yourself by using statements like "I RELEASE THE BELIEF THAT I AM UNLOVABLE."

"I RELEASE" is a very powerful (and positively stated) instruction to the subconscious. Then, reprogramming with typical positive affirmations like "I AM LOVABLE, LOVING, AND LOVED" can be effective.

Self-Worth and the Solar Plexus Chakra

In the last chapter, we talked about the importance of the aura and chakras in healing major blockages. We also spoke of ways that remedies and work on the energy body complement each other. Those who are not familiar with that concept and who skipped that section may wish to go back to it, as we will refer to the chakras repeatedly in the chapters that follow.

The solar plexus chakra, located below the heart and just above the waist, is the seat of self-worth, self-esteem, confidence, and the self-concept. Although all chakras continue to evolve throughout life, each has a period of emphasis during child development. The solar plexus predominates during toddler and preschool years. It's natural for young children to be self-involved, because it's an important developmental task to come to know who you are, separate from those around you. A healthy solar plexus grows from the attention and even the adoration we get from our parents, grandparents, aunts, uncles, and other adults when we are young. Poor solar plexus development results in low self-esteem or even narcissism, both of which powerfully affect our confidence, capacity for self-expression, and relationships.

Low self-esteem is common among those who grow up in dysfunctional families. The solar plexus energy the child does receive can be less than wholesome. Addiction is hard on the self-worth of the addict, so the solar plexus is damaged. There is also a spillover effect, in that the more damaged the next-door heart center is from drinking, the less effectively the solar plexus functions. Many alcoholics are grandiose when they are drinking, then depressed and self-hating when they're not. The child may imitate this pattern, alternating between grandiosity and depression.

The solar plexus goes through another crucial refinement during adolescence. An important task of this period is to establish an identity among peers and to figure out who you are, separate from your family. Authoritarian, rejecting parents make this task difficult, as do merging parents who have boundary problems. More difficult still is being different from peers and rejected by them, since gaining a sense of belonging is another important task. Children from dysfunctional homes are already different and also may not have learned certain social skills. Self-concepts formed during the teens tend to persist and to affect how attractive and love-worthy we feel. It may be necessary to work on clearing out the damage done at this age.

Even in adulthood, a major failure such as being fired or a love rejection can also damage the solar plexus and self-esteem, so healing may be required.

Tools for Healing the Solar Plexus

One key to change is to repair the solar plexus through a variety of tools, especially in combination with the essences given earlier. Sunflower, in particular, is good for the solar plexus. If you like crystals, you might tape citrine or other yellow stones on the area, being sure to cleanse them extensively afterwards. Energy work methods like Reiki and MariEL are especially useful when directed at the solar plexus. I also find that Earthfriends' Inner Sun oil penetrates deeply into the solar plexus and stimulates healing.

In combination with remedies like Sunflower or Buttercup, light work on the solar plexus is also helpful. By this we mean the kind of light present in the aura. It isn't necessary to visualize light in order for it to be effective; the Higher Self knows how to do it. Imagine a swirling ball of multicolored light in your solar plexus. As it swirls, notice which colors the solar plexus seems most hungry for. Repeat the meditation later with a pure light of that color. Or, if you wish, finish up with that color during this session.

Another exercise with light is particularly relevant to self-worth problems coming from the way your parents dealt with you. Imagine yourself safe and cozy in a bubble of white light. Imagine someone who has damaged your self-esteem—family members, lovers, bosses, even friends—in another bubble. Now pretend their bubble has a huge magnet on the front, and it is pulling out of your solar plexus their judgment, condemnation, or rejection. When that pull has gone on for a while, move the bubble behind you, where the magnet will draw out energy you have psychically absorbed. You may find the pull even stronger there. Then move it back in front again.

Finally, imagine a magnet on the front of your bubble that draws back all the power you have given others. To finish, dissolve both bubbles. When early conditions are involved, it may be useful to go through the exercise year by year, beginning inside the womb, up to the present. Mullein, for being true to yourself, and Sagebrush, for letting go of false influences or self-concepts, would be especially good remedies to use with this exercise.

Remedies to Help Change Narcissism

Self-absorption is not a sign of excess ego, but rather of energy hung up in the solar plexus so that the ego needs constant reassurance and attention. When true pride in one's gifts and accomplishment is present, little validation is required. When it is not present, no amount of stroking from the outside can fill the void.

Yellow Cone Flower, described earlier, is useful in letting go of the need for excess stroking.

Narcissism easily comes into the picture when both the solar plexus and the heart chakras are constricted. Therefore, both chakras may need to be cleared and strengthened for a healthy, balanced ego. Tools and remedies for the heart chakra are given in chapter 8.

There are essences to counteract self-obsession. You and I don't need them, of course, but, boy, do we know some people we'd love to give them to! Many are the same as for low self-esteem, since remedies often serve to balance either extreme.

Sunflower, so important for people with low self-esteem, also helps those who are too egotistical.

Bach's Heather is for self-centered people who are wrapped up in their own troubles.

Bach's Chicory can also be useful for people who need to be the center of attention, even in negative ways.

Trillium is another useful antidote. FES says it leads to selflessness, working for the common good, and sacrifice of personal desires.

Their Star Thistle is described as developing the qualities of sharing, generosity, and giving of oneself to others, especially where there has been an inability to share oneself or one's possessions.

Finally, their Larkspur replaces self-aggrandizement with generosity and altruism.

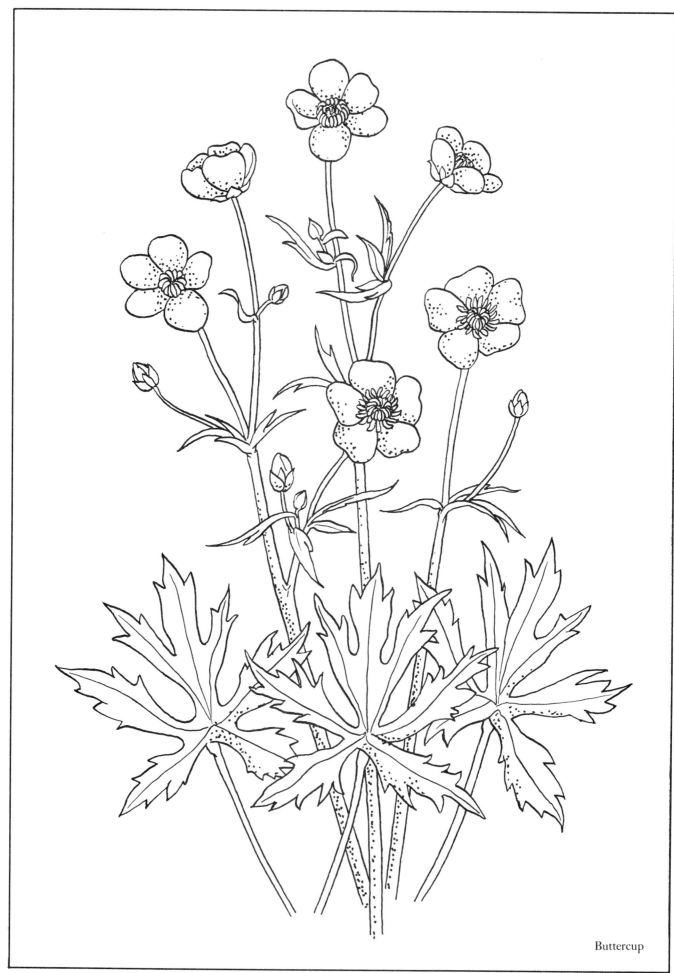

Buttercup

BUTTERCUP

Aliases: Latin name *ranunculus*, meaning "little frog," because of its preference for wet habitats. Also known as crowfoot, because the leaves resemble crow's feet, as gold knots, and as "crazy," because the plant was thought to cause madness.

Companies making the essence: Bailey, FES, Pegasus.

Essence qualities: The FES description say it is excellent for valuing your own gifts and appreciating your own worth. It is recommended for those who tend to undervalue their life-style or vocation, who do not feel good enough, or are shy.

Lore: Some believe they are the lilies of the field mentioned in the Bible, which outshone King Solomon. Irish farmers rubbed the blossoms on their cows' udders at May Day in the belief that it increased the production of milk. Children were told to hold a buttercup under their chin. If a yellow reflection appeared, it was proof they loved butter. Birthday flower for September 18. In the language of flowers, it conveyed the message "You are radiant with charms."

What the plant is like: These small, golden-yellow perennials look as though they've just been dipped in melted butter. The dark, waxy, green foliage stands about 2″ (5 cm) tall, with five-petaled blooms about an inch across. There are about forty species in North America, with many of these varieties originally imported from Europe. Some species grow from bulblike roots called corms, others from runners like strawberries, and others from seeds. They open and close with the sun, being open from sunrise to sunset, but not on rainy days.

Uses: Not for eating—livestock avoid them because of their acrid taste. In homeopathic dilution, use for bad effects of alcohol, delirium tremens, and shingles.

Reflections: Their reliance on sunlight for opening and closing suggests an association with the solar plexus and with divine light. The shiny bright yellow color induces calmness, joy, and mental stimulation. The homeopathic association with the effects of alcohol suggests it may help recovering alcoholics get back their self-worth.

Affirmations: I RELEASE THE BELIEF THAT I'M NOT GOOD ENOUGH.

I LOVE AND APPRECIATE MY DIVINELY GIVEN TALENTS.

I VALUE MY CONTRIBUTIONS EQUALLY WITH ALL OTHERS.

Astrological correlations: Strengthens the Sun, which governs self-expression, and any planets in the fifth house, which shows the ways we are creative.

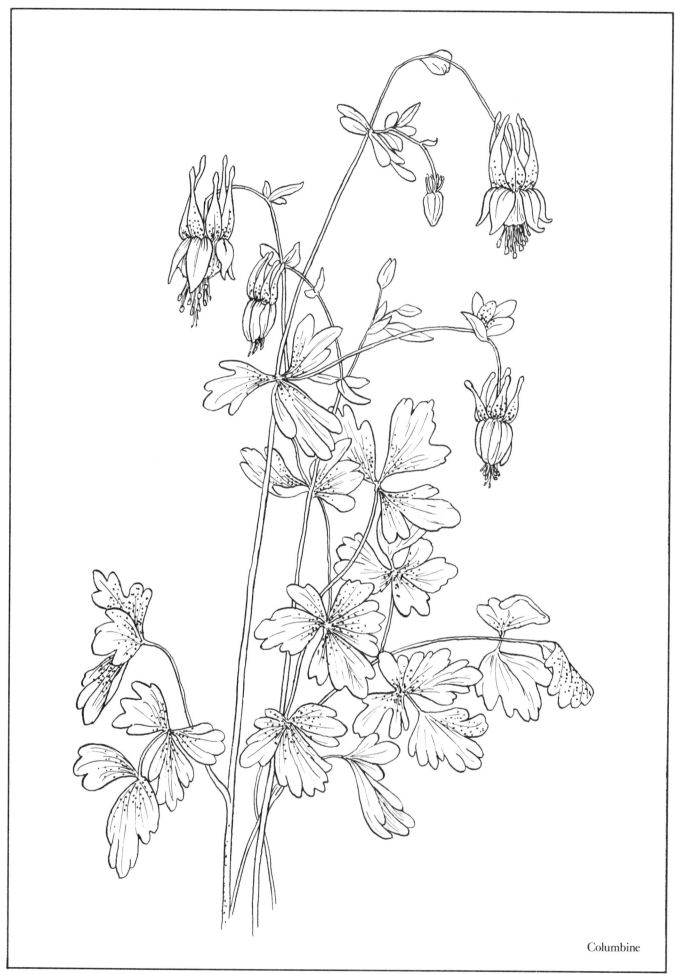

Columbine

COLUMBINE

Aliases: Latin name *Aquilegia canadensis*. *Canadensis*, from Canada and *aquilegia* from the Latin word *aquila*, for eagle, since the base of the flower resembles an eagle's claw. Common names include granny's bonnets and lion's herb.

Companies making the essence: The Alaskan Flower Essence Project, FES, Pegasus.

Essence qualities: The Alaskan catalog says it is for self-appreciation and appreciation of your unique and personal beauty, regardless of how it differs from others.

Lore: The name comes from the Italian word for dove, *columbina*, because it reminded people of a dove drinking at a fountain or spring. Italians use *columbina* as a term of endearment for sweethearts, especially the sweet, virginal type. As a love potion, the seeds were crushed and rubbed on the body. Native American men smoked wild columbine seeds with tobacco for luck before calling on a favorite lady friend. In the language of flowers, it meant folly or an abandoned lover. However, a purple columbine carried the message "I am resolved to win," while a red one meant "anxious and trembling." In religious circles, because the word means dove, the flower also came to represent the holy spirit and thus it appeared symbolically in paintings. Colorado state flower.

What the plant is like: The plant grows up to 2' (60 cm), with showy, nodding blossoms of various colors, up to 2" (5 cm) across. The flowers hang downwards, with five spurs on each blossom. Bumblebees and hummingbirds visit for the nectar. This slender, hardy perennial blooms from mid-spring to early summer. It is a member of the buttercup family, although there is little resemblance.

Uses: Herbalists boiled the roots and leaves for tea, using it for everything from scurvy and the plague to fever and bladder trouble. To ease labor pains, they mixed the seeds with wine. Homeopathically, it is used for hysteria and dysmenorrhea.

Reflections: I use this often for self-esteem. It might also be effective for those who continually compare themselves to others.

Affirmations: I CHERISH MY OWN SPECIAL BEAUTY.

I EMBRACE MY DIFFERENCES AND APPRECIATE MY WORTH.

I RELEASE ALL COMPARISONS OF MYSELF WITH OTHERS.

Astrological correlations: Helpful for difficult Venus aspects, especially to Uranus. Strengthening to the Sun in all difficult aspects, especially Sun/Uranus or Aquarian placements.

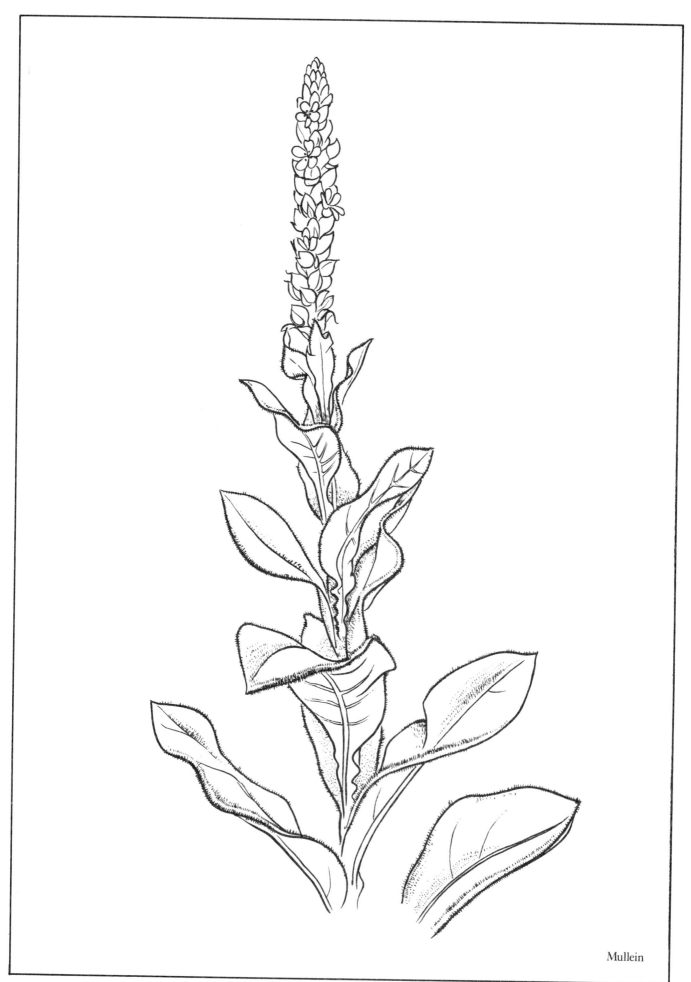

Mullein

MULLEIN

Aliases: Latin name *Verbascum thapsus*. *Verbascum* comes from the Latin word *barbātus*, meaning bearded; Thapsus was a town in Tunisia. The large variety of common names included Aaron's rod, hag's tapers, candlestick plant, graveyard dust, and Our Lady's candle.

Companies making the essence: Desert Alchemy, FES, Pegasus.

Essence qualities: FES says it is for being true to oneself; fulfillment of one's true potential; listening to one's own inner guidance; developing an inner sense of morality and values.

Lore: It was dipped in suet and burned as a torch in outdoor religious ceremonies, both Christian and pre-Christian, hence the common names. (Hag's tapers referred to witches.) Mullein was widely believed in Europe and the East to repel evil spirits, so monasteries grew it to protect against the devil. People hung it indoors at home to keep negativity away and stuffed it in pillows to guard against nightmares.

What the plant is like: A tall biennial. The first year, it is a rosette of large, pale or white, woolly leaves lying next to the ground. The second year, a stalk up to 4′ (1.2 m) tall grows from the center of this rosette with a dense spike of yellow or pale five-petaled flowers. It grows on dry banks and wastelands in a temperate climate and flowers in July.

Uses: Widely used by Native Americans as a cold remedy and against mumps. Herbalists recommend it for infectious diseases like tuberculosis and to soothe the kidneys and swollen joints. It was also a remedy for gout and was considered a natural pain reliever without any habit-forming properties. The crushed leaves were used to remove warts and to relieve hemorrhoids. The leaves are a natural source of iron, magnesium, potassium, and sulfur. Farmers gave it to cows for respiratory problems and to horses after shoeing, to heal their hooves.

Reflections: The description seems to be stated positively in terms of paying attention to your own counsel and being true to yourself, while the lore suggests it was a protection against negative interference by spirits. I have found it helpful with people who are groping to find their purpose in life.

Affirmations: I RESPECT AND AM GUIDED BY MY HIGHER SELF.
THE PATH TO MY HIGHEST POTENTIAL IS CLEARLY MARKED.

Astrological correlations: When the Sun in the birth chart forms an angle to the planet Uranus, these individuals may need Mullein in order to value their differentness. Other possibilities would be Uranus in the twelfth house or when Uranus forms few aspects to other planets.

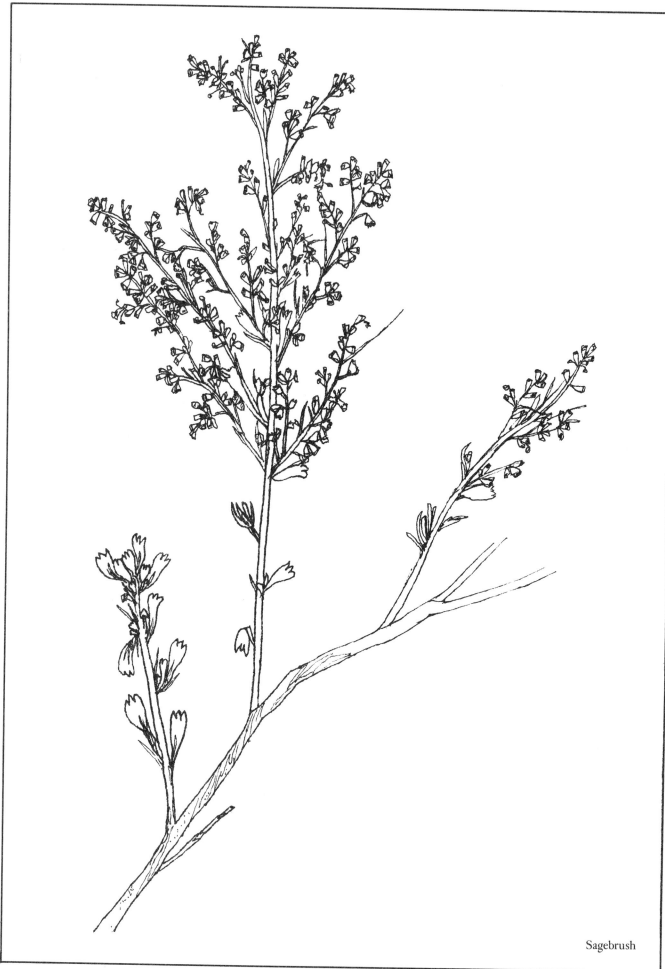

Sagebrush

SAGEBRUSH

Aliases: Latin name *Artemisia tridentata*. *Artemisia*, for the goddess Artemis, or Diana. *Tridentata* means (leaves) having three teeth.

Companies making the essence: Desert Alchemy, FES, Pegasus.

Essence qualities: FES recommends it for letting go of false self-images that no longer serve a productive purpose, being true to the essential self, and for offsetting false identification and influences. Matt Wood gives an excellent analysis of the remedy in *Seven Herbs*, recommending it for those caught in no-win situations.

Lore: Sagebrush was a very holy herb to Native Americans, who burned it to purify and cleanse negativity. It was especially used in the purifying sweat lodges. Students of shamanism still use it today to clear vibrations. State flower of Nevada.

What the plant is like: Sagebrush is a member of the Artemisia Family of plants, which includes wormwood and mugwort. Many of these plants grow in the desert or very dry areas. The fine, grey, velvety hairs protect the plant from the harsh sun. The foliage is highly pungent and the taste is sharp.

Uses: The plant was valued by the Native Americans of the Northwest as a poultice for wounds and rashes, and as a hot decoction for colds. It was considered a good tonic for stomach ailments and indigestion, and to rinse the mouth after eating to prevent bad breath. As a hot poultice, it was applied to the forehead to relieve migraines.

Reflections: I have found it excellent for the upwardly mobile, who have to reconcile their new status in the world with their origins. These folks often struggle with sadness and even guilt at being more successful than their families. It is especially good for upwardly mobile minority group members.

Affirmations: THAT WHICH IS NOT ME, I WILLINGLY RELEASE.

I LET GO OF OUTGROWN IDEAS ABOUT MYSELF.

I FACE AND LOVINGLY ACCEPT MY TRUE SELF.

Astrological correlations: It strengthens the Sun, especially when the rising sign is incompatible with the true nature.

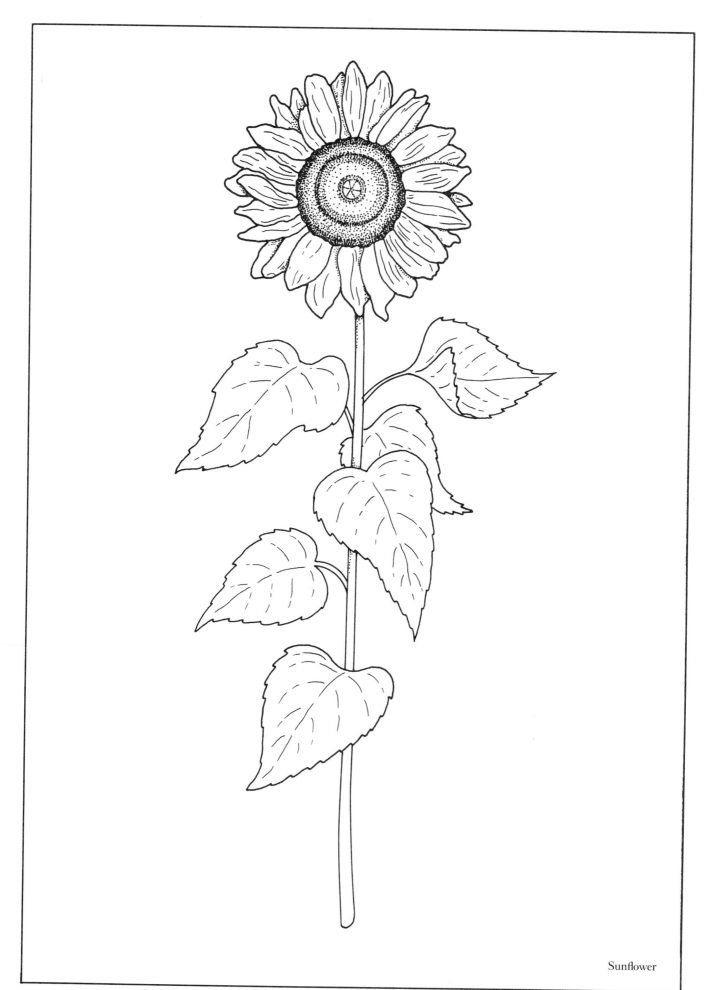

Sunflower

SUNFLOWER

Aliases: Latin name *Helianthus annuus*. *Hēlios* means sun, *anthos* means flower, and *annuus* denotes an annual. Common names were marigold of Peru and Indian sun.

Companies making the essence: Alaskan Flower Essence Project, FES, Harebell, Pegasus.

Essence qualities: FES says it balances ego, expression of individuality, and conflict relating to parents, especially the father. Distortion in the ego, whether from low self-esteem or vanity.

Lore: The sunflower was venerated by sun worshippers, including the Incas and Native North Americans. Women who wished to conceive ate the seeds. In the language of flowers, denoted haughtiness. Birthday flower for June 30 and state flower for Kansas.

It was long believed that sunflowers turn their heads, east to west, in the course of the day, to follow the sun's path. Some busy botanist photographed them all day long and proved to his satisfaction that this is not true. Another myth debunked by science! However, veteran gardener Louise Riotte notes that only young plants turn their heads.

What the plant is like: An annual, blooming late summer to early fall, the sunflower stands 3' to 12' (.9 to 3.6 m), on a rough, hairy stem. The flowers are up to 6″ (15 cm) across. The large center disk, where the seeds grow, is made of tiny brown or yellow flowers, and yellow petals ray outward from the disk. They need full sunlight and protection against the wind. When fields are abandoned, the sunflower is among the first plants to grow. It releases toxins into the soil that inhibit other plants from growing nearby, even its own offspring.

Uses: The seeds are edible, and they can be made into cereal, flour, soap, or oil. A form of coffee can be brewed from the hulls. The stalks can be ground into fodder and have even been used to make cloth and a substitute for tobacco. The seeds are an important food for birds.

Reflections: Though the biggest and the showiest flower in the garden, the sunflower plant is important only for its seeds. We, too, may strive to be important, but in the long run only our contributions will last.

Affirmations: I AM A CHILD OF GOD AND AM WORTHY OF LOVE.

I VALUE MY OWN CONTRIBUTIONS AND THOSE OF ALL OTHERS.

I AM AT ONCE CONFIDENT AND HUMBLE.

Astrological correlations: Sunflower strengthens the Sun in any horoscope. Leos seem to need this remedy—whether Leo Sun, Moon, or rising sign.

Self-Esteem—The Foundation of a Better Life

There is good reason why an entire chapter has been devoted to self-esteem. When people are consumed with self-hate or troubled with self-doubt, their hard work and efforts often meet with frustration. They tend to sabotage themselves unconsciously or, at the very least, to present themselves in ways that keep others from taking them seriously. Low self-esteem can also either twist relationships or make it hard to attract them in the first place. When you stand in a loving relationship to yourself, you will be kind and gentle with yourself in other healing work. The underlying belief that you are okay gives you enough confidence to face tough emotions or memories that often surface in the course of such healing. You will be coming from a place of strength.

In moving through the work in this book, if you ever doubt you can do it, or if you begin to blame yourself for your shortcomings, go back to the remedies and other tools discussed in this chapter.

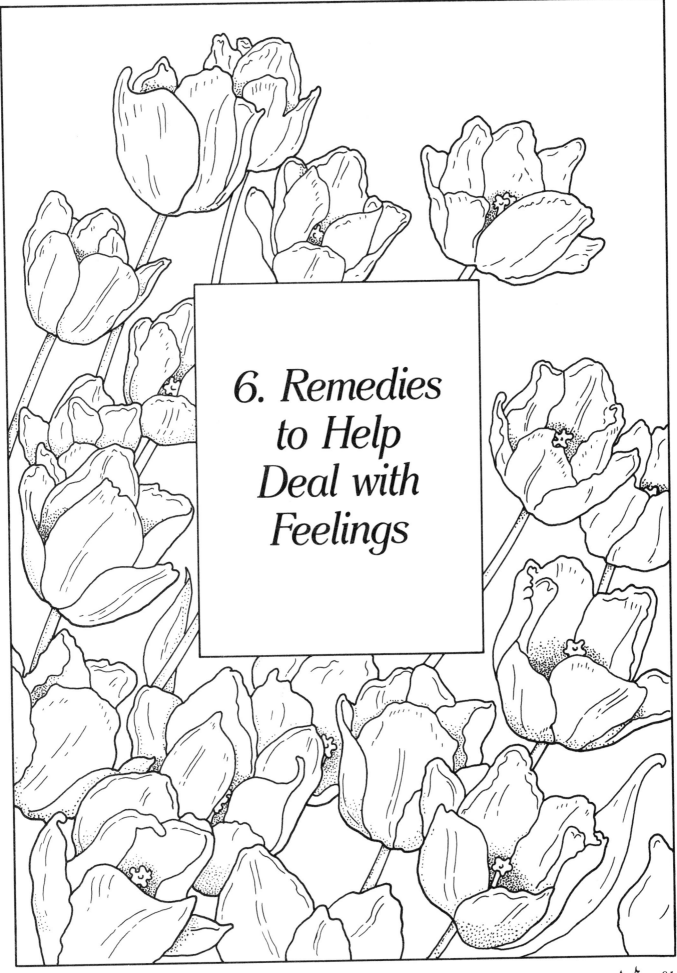

6. Remedies to Help Deal with Feelings

Understanding and dealing with emotions is a lifelong task, and our society and upbringing give little assistance with it. People are rewarded for suppressing emotions and subtly or not so subtly dissuaded from fully experiencing or expressing them. This cultural prohibition is one reason for the increase in addictions, the widespread feeling of alienation, and the high incidence of depression.

Any time we are out of touch with the healthy and normal signals from the center of our being, we are likely to make mistakes and poor choices. When we lose touch with ourselves, then our behavior in relationships, social contacts, and career is based on false premises. Self-esteem can suffer from disowning such vital parts of our nature— "If my feelings are bad and unacceptable, I must be bad too." When strong emotions are repressed long enough, they may come out in other ways— often distorted and undesirable ways—including malfunctions in our bodies, habits, or relationships.

Flower remedies help us to understand these signals as they arise and to work them through without getting stuck. Remedies also help release of emotional blockages that have accumulated. Again, this is not to suggest that they can replace needed therapy or healing, but they speed the process and result in more conscious awareness. The gift of the remedies, as opposed to therapy alone, is that you more quickly become accepting of the full range of emotional responses and thus are less likely to hold on to or bury them.

With essences, we have a tool for handling feelings so they do not accumulate but are dealt with in mature, conscious ways. We don't vent them in a wholesome or inappropriate fashion, but we don't cut them off either. We will discuss remedies for fear, anxiety, guilt, resentment, anger, depression, and grief. We will pinpoint remedies that can be helpful in an emotional crisis and several that make it easier to face and deal with feelings.

First, Know What You're Feeling

In a culture that rewards repression, it is not always easy to know what we really feel. Thus, the first step may be to reclaim these disowned reactions and become comfortable with them.

For people who live in their heads and are dominated by intellect, Australian Bush Flower Essences' Isopogon leads to more connection with the heart and feelings.

Bach's Clematis is for space cadets who all too often drift off into a dream world in order not to feel anything.

Bach's Agrimony is recommended for people who put up a cheerful front, but behind it are tortured by painful emotions and memories. Many practitioners, including Dr. Bach himself, have noted that it is good for alcoholism. My recovering clients have often benefited from it, because they previously had used substances to hide from their real feelings. (A profile of this intriguing herb appears at the end of the chapter.)

In chapter 4, we focused on remedies to enhance psychotherapy, discussing preparations for dealing with and sorting out emotions. The ones in that chapter can help even if you aren't in therapy and are just working on your own. Here, however, it is important to remind you of three indispensable essences by FES that were discussed in that chapter—Scarlet Monkeyflower, Black-eyed Susan, and Fuchsia. Chapter 4 gives hints on how to decide which of these three is most appropriate.

Scarlet Monkeyflower gives the courage to face or express powerful emotions, especially when there is repression or fear of intense responses that may show up in hidden or abrupt ways.

Black-eyed Susan, which brings insight when there is resistance to looking at emotions, will be profiled here.

Fuchsia allows greater awareness of repressed or deep-seated reactions that are often expressed as hyperemotionality and psychosomatic illness. It can be a cathartic leading to release.

Desert Alchemy's Emotional Awareness Formula allows you to feel without judging, needing to control with your mind, or blocking.

Where subconscious states erupt in uncontrolled and even irresponsible ways, their Ocotillo encourages understanding and acceptance.

FES's Deer Brush brings greater awareness of underlying and unconscious motives, so that you may become more honest and open.

Illyarrie, an Australian remedy made by Living Essences, helps those impasses where you want to avoid the pain of dealing with something.

Once you're able to feel your emotions, however, you don't want to hold on to them. Again, Scarlet Monkeyflower, Fuchsia, and perhaps Yerba Santa can facilitate working them through.

FES's Chamomile calms people who are upset and, taken over time, builds an inner serenity.

Chaparral is a key remedy for releasing emotions and gaining insight into them, especially through dreams.

Along with the remedies given above, you may want to work with affirmations. You could repeat the following in the Sondra Ray manner of 70 times 7, or you might design some that are more specific to your own patterns:

I RELEASE THE FEAR OF
EXPERIENCING MY TRUE FEELINGS.

I EMBRACE MY FEELINGS AND DEAL
WITH THEM CONSCIOUSLY.

MY FEELINGS ARE APPROPRIATELY
AND SAFELY EXPRESSED.

Layers of the Onion

In chapter 3 we spoke about the process of essence work, in which it is typical for one layer after another to emerge, like peeling an onion. Nowhere is the onion metaphor more true than in responses that mask deeper feelings. The rage-aholic, for instance, may be covering up terror or sadness. The person who is consumed with guilt may use it as a defense against a sense of powerlessness. The chronically anxious may use anxiety to hold down anger. Our most frequent and consuming emotions are often catchall defenses against a range of other states of mind we find less acceptable.

In chapter 2, talking about how remedies work, we learned that our most characteristic emotions are habitual. I have often noticed that we each have a set of response habits based on feelings that our parents and others who were important to us said were okay or not-okay. In order to please them, we began as children to convert the not-okay reactions into ones that were more acceptable to them. In some families, anger was taboo, but depression was rewarded by extra attention. In others, crying was punished or shamed, while ag-

gressiveness was admired. Others learned to diffuse (and defuse!) difficult emotions by going into a passive, helpless, confused state.

You may already have an idea of your own set of emotional habits that cover up other responses you don't know what to do with. Or, you may come to know them through self-observation, especially in the course of taking remedies. In particular, as you take mixtures for some of your catchall responses, the next layer of underlying feelings will come to the surface.

For some women, these habitual states often come on strongly during the premenstrual phase. We tend to put them down as trivial. "Oh, you're just getting your period." However, the feelings arising during that phase are our *real* feelings, even though they're somewhat exaggerated for being suppressed all month. We cannot ignore them if we wish to be healthy. Taking remedies regularly during this phase will pave the way for dealing with our lives in new and healthier ways. Rather than an aggravating inconvenience, these cyclical reactions can be signals that lead us to greater wholeness.

Coping with Crisis

Remedies can be especially helpful during periods of crisis. Emergency essence combinations are made by a variety of companies, and generally one is sufficient for your repertoire. I myself use two with clients and can't yet see any difference between them. However, my pendulum does, sometimes recommending one, sometimes the other, and occasionally both together or in succession. They are Rescue Remedy by Bach and Emergency Essence by the Australian Bush Essences. Another is Desert Alchemy's Emergency Essence, which is said to carry with it the sense of *emerg*ing through the crisis.

It is a truism that inherent in crisis is the possibility of change and growth. Essences facilitate using crisis for insight and evolution. Taken every few hours, the essences also maintain calmness and clarity during the emergency and make it possible to throw off the aftereffects more quickly. Therefore, it would be useful to continue them for a while after the threat is over. Generally, you are to take them full strength during the entire period, except, of course, for recovering alcoholics, who might find the brandy solvent too stressful at such times.

We've spoken before about Rescue Remedy, a Bach classic available even in health food stores that don't carry the entire set. I was once out walking with a friend who is deathly allergic to bee stings. She was wearing sandals, and a bee stung her on the toe. By some "coincidence," I was carrying Rescue Remedy in my bag and applied it to the sting. She was amazed, not to mention relieved, to find she had no allergic reaction at all.

Rescue Remedy is excellent in physical as well as emotional crisis. It is extremely beneficial taken in the few days before and after surgery, cutting down on the shock and speeding recovery. Gregory Vlamis' book, *Flowers to the Rescue*, mentioned earlier, is full of case histories supplied by physicians, veterinarians, and other health professionals about Rescue Remedy's uses.[1] It is an important addition to any first-aid kit.

Living Essences of Australia features Flag Flower that helps to calm people who fear they are going to have a nervous breakdown.

This sounds similar to Bach's Cherry Plum, one of the ingredients in Rescue Remedy. Used separately, Cherry Plum relieves the fear that you may lose control, go crazy, and hurt yourself or others.

I have often given FES's Red Clover to people who are upset about someone else's upheaval. The catalog describes it as providing centeredness during states of emergency or emotionally charged family situations. When others are hysterical, it fosters the stability to stay centered.

Facing and Overcoming Fear and Anxiety

Many people are plagued by fears of one sort or another. Fear makes every effort more difficult: we often waste precious energy worrying about things that never happen. I remember going through a very anxious time, when every day or two a new worry would become my total reality. Someone suggested I make a worry box, writing my concern down on a piece of paper, praying over it, and then placing it inside the box for God to take care of. After six weeks, I opened the box to find 26 slips of paper. Only one of the things I was so concerned about had actually happened. This realization helped me stop worrying so much.

Essences can also help correct the fear habit. Number one for this purpose is Bach's Mimulus, for fear of something specific, or of many specific things, as well as more general timidity and shyness. I generally combine it with other remedies specifically related to the situation.

Add Money Plant if the concerns are financial.

Borage is a wonderful remedy that FES says is for "cheerful courage." The very idea of cheerful courage is heartening, somehow. One of borage's common names was herb of gladness: the Greeks used it in wine to give a feeling of well-being. Cordials made from it were used to cheer up those suffering from such prolonged illnesses as tuberculosis.

FES also suggests Garlic for releasing fear, insecurities, and nervousness such as stage fright.

There are a variety of preparations for terror or panic, including Bach's Rock Rose, Australian Bush Flower Essences' Grey Spider Flower, and Living Essences' Pink Fairies. (Rock Rose is a component of Rescue Remedy.) They are helpful in emergencies or life-threatening situations, of course, but such events rarely confront us in our daily lives. However, should you be tested by having to make a speech, audition for a part, or take an actual examination, you'll find that they will restore calmness so that you can function to the best of your abilities.

While living in California, I had to take a state licensing exam, although I had received my degree in social work long before and had many years of experience. The test included a variety of long-forgotten theories, newer additions to the curriculum, and social welfare laws of the State of California. The oral section involved being questioned by a panel of hard-nosed examiners. I was terrified. Just before going into the room, I took a dose of Rock Rose straight from the stock bottle and immediately felt cool and collected. I passed, too, even though the majority of candidates have to repeat the testing process twice or more! A good income undoubtedly awaits the person who gets the Rock Rose concession for license examination candidates.

In recovery, the alcoholic or other addicted person may undergo panic attacks. These are a phase in the process of clearing the energy body of damage done by the addiction. Thus, along with health care and essences such as Rock Rose or Rescue Remedy, the recovering individual with anxiety attacks might want energy work like Reiki, MariEl, or Jin Shin Jyutsu. Such supports also would help anyone who is suffering from anxiety or the aftereffects of a shock, trauma, or other emergency.

Many times, however, people have the uncomfortable experience of being nervous and fearful with no clear-cut reason. If you're anxious and don't know why, Bach's Aspen may very well reveal what you're actually upset about. Anxiety is a generalized response through which the unconscious masks feelings the person finds unacceptable, like anger or sexual attraction. It is also one of the symptoms of serious depression, so if you have recurrent or severe anxiety, consult a physician.

The legends about aspen are revealing. The medieval church taught that the cross was made of aspen and so it trembles, out of guilt. One study showed that people who have something on their conscience are more fearful. No doubt the unconscious anticipates and even desires punishment for its transgressions. This arises both because of childhood experiences of discipline and because the Higher Self wants us to grow and evolve into better people. Therefore, when guilt is an underlying cause of anxiety, Aspen may bring that layer of feelings to the surface, to be dealt with.

Toxic Shame and Self-Hate

Flower essences can be a major aid in dealing with toxic shame.

Australian Bush Flower Essences suggests Billy Goat Plum for self-loathing.

Among the Bach remedies, Crab Apple is helpful to the client consumed with self-loathing and shame, while Holly is the antidote to self-hate.

Beech, by Bach, is more often given to those who are critical and judgmental of others. However, at the root of this behavior is often a person who is excessively self-critical. I've often had good results using Beech with those who are too hard on themselves.

I've also had excellent results with The Alaskan Flower Essence Project's Columbine, recommended for an appreciation of one's unique and personal beauty. (Columbine is also profiled later.)

Alpine Azalea is an excellent essence for living in total acceptance of yourself.

The Australian company Living Essences offers Correa to release dissatisfaction with ourselves and to accept our shortcomings.

There are a number of fine possibilities, so I generally haul them all out of the box and let the pendulum indicate which ones to use.

Guilt and Resentment—The Siamese Twins

The topic of guilt could easily have been included in the chapter on self-esteem, because it can make us hate ourselves. Likewise, essences for shame discussed there, Crab Apple, for example, might also be tested for people who are troubled with remorse for past deeds.

A primary remedy for guilt is Pine, by Bach. Profiled later, pine is often an ingredient in household cleaning products. To many of us, a house that smells of pine seems like a truly clean house. Likewise, cleansing ourselves of guilt can be an effect of Pine essence.

Although we try to find something in the present to fasten this unpleasant feeling onto, very often the chronically guilty have a kind of existential guilt, not about anything particular, just guilt on the hoof. One woman, a hard worker in a service field, was conscientiously honest in every way. Nonetheless, she was so guilt-ridden that when a police car drove by, she cringed and had a dramatic surge of fear that they were coming for her. When she went into a store carrying something in her purse that the store sold, she was anxious the whole time that they would think she was shoplifting. After several months on Pine, she was free of this lifelong burden of neurotic guilt and could laugh at her former behavior. Furthermore, she had been very much the unwise rescuer type, taken advantage of by people who played on her sympathy. After Pine, she could no longer be manipulated by guilt trips. "Now," she says, "I only respond to genuine need."

The remedies are a highly spiritualizing force. If you take them over a period of time, you change how you operate. With Pine, for example, when you've done something you aren't proud of, you are able to make amends, learn from the experience, and become a better person. Previously you might have eaten yourself up with guilt, too ashamed to do anything about it.

Part of the healing may involve the need to make a formal karmic housecleaning. It may be instructive to read the chapters about Steps Eight and Nine in the Alcoholics Anonymous book *Twelve Steps and Twelve Traditions*. Step Eight says, "Made a list of all persons we had harmed and became willing to make amends to them," while Step Nine says, "Made direct amends to such people wherever possible, except when to do so would injure them or others." Even if you are one of the rare individuals who doesn't fit into any of the plethora of 12-step programs, the process outlined for these two steps could foster a deep healing. There is great wisdom in the spiritual path involved with the steps.

One of my therapy clients was a recovering alcoholic who, through self-centeredness and worse, had hurt many people in the depths of his disease. Even in recovery, his self-esteem remained very low—he says it was down around his ankles. A combination of Pine and Crab Apple helped him to muster the strength to move forward on Steps Eight and Nine. When he made amends, the responses were much more positive than if he'd approached people with the combination of guilt and self-justification he was feeling before. This is just one example of how flower remedies and recovery programs can work together. People in twelve-step programs who would like to use remedies to help them work the steps may read "Remedies for Recovery" in the Appendix.

There is nothing more corrosive to happiness—or to relationships—than bitterness and resentment. No one voluntarily stays around a bitter individual for very long. This habit—I repeat, habit—drives people away and results in more and more isolation.

Willow, by Bach, is an extremely important remedy for resentment. When it goes even deeper, into hatred and vengefulness, their Holly may also be crucial. (Willow is profiled at the end of this chapter, and Holly in chapter 4.)

Also beneficial is Alaskan Flower Essence Project's Fireweed, for releasing old angers.

Their Mountain Wormwood is an important essence for unforgiven areas in the self or others.

Australian Bush Flower Essences features Dagger Hakea for resentment and bitterness toward close family, friends, or lovers, leading to forgiveness.

Their Mountain Devil, like Holly, is said to heal hatred, jealousy, suspicion, and other barriers to love, leading to unconditional love.

Accepting and Releasing Anger

Learning to deal with anger as it arises prevents the accumulation of resentment. When you clear the energy body of old anger, especially through a combination of remedies and energy work, you don't have a backlog to be triggered by every irritation. Bodywork may also be important for moving anger held in the physical body.

In addition, the Alaskan Flower Essence Project's Fireweed is excellent for healing old angers. Steve Johnson, one of the founders, points out that fireweed grows profusely in areas burnt by forest fires, where it is the first plant to come back.[2] Also test the remedies for resentment listed above.

A form of therapy useful in preventing future buildups is assertiveness training, which gives you the tools to deal with aggravating situations more effectively. Assertiveness is not about aggressiveness, but rather about setting boundaries and having the ability to negotiate in conflict. We do not generally acquire these skills as we grow up, but we can learn them. There are two especially good essences to go with assertiveness training.

Harebell's Snapdragon is a throat chakra remedy that frees the person to speak up about negative feelings. Irritation in the throat or voice is an indication that you might need it.

FES's Trumpet Vine also helps you speak out. (Again, you would see the signature in the megaphone-shaped blossom.)

We noted before how the bright red color of Scarlet Monkeyflower is an indication of its special relationship to facing and dealing with anger. It is not to be neglected in working with this emotion. Interestingly, when you look at the Latin names on the bottle, Scarlet Monkeyflower is a member of the *mimulus* family, along with Sticky Monkeyflower, a remedy for intimacy. Remember, however, that Mimulus itself is for fear and timidity. Curious! No doubt, it is only as fear is relieved that an individual feels safe both to be intimate and to express angry feelings in close relationships. Studying botanical families and Latin names gives many such insights into connections between essences.

Both Mimulus and Scarlet Monkeyflower are red and will be recognized by the astrologically sophisticated as related to the red planet Mars.

Some people are constitutionally more irritable than others; this is apparent even in babies. (In fact, if irritable babies were treated with remedies, their lives and their parents would be more peaceful.) Bach's Impatiens is well tested for impatient, fast-moving and -thinking people who get annoyed at slower ones. My Aries clients almost always seem to need Impatiens. Aries, of course, is ruled by Mars, and another dynamic of this planet is that it is related both to anger and to energy. It is well known that fatigue is often tied to suppressed anger. In fact, people who take remedies for fatigue, like Bach's Olive or Hornbeam, sometime go through a period of irritability as they build up renewed energy. Likewise, overtired children—and adults—can be cranky. It might be a good thing to test irritable clients for the fatigue essences.

More extreme reactions, like outbursts of rage, can be softened by Cherry Plum. It benefits those who are afraid to confront anger because of fear they will lose control and hurt someone. One recovering alcoholic I worked with in therapy had been sober in A.A. for five years and was still punching holes in walls. He no longer punched holes in people, as he once did, but he still found it a strain to keep his anger under control once aroused. After taking just one bottle of Cherry Plum as a single remedy, he was able to excuse himself and go for a walk when a situation came up that once would have made him explode. After he had cooled down, he would come back and talk it out. This remarkable progress was not explained by any other change in his treatment or recovery program.

Some Thoughts About Depression and the Remedies

Many people say they are depressed when really they mean they are sad. The word "depression" is both overused and misused, and it is important to distinguish between its popular connotation and actual clinical depression, which requires medical treatment. There are two kinds of clinical depression: *chronic depression* and *reactive depression*.

Chronic depression often results from a biochemical abnormality or an extremely difficult situation that has lasted for many years. *Reactive depression* is temporary and related to some recent loss. For instance, you can experience reactive depression when a loved one dies, a marriage or other love relationship breaks up, when you lose your job or retire, or when the children move out.

Clinical depression wears many masks other than sadness. They include fatigue, hopelessness, purposelessness, lack of interest in sex or other pleasures, major weight losses or gains, irritability, sleeplessness or sleeping too much, and suicidal impulses. Many addictions, especially to alcohol or sugar, are an attempt to self-medicate depression. In fact, geneticists have isolated genes involved in biochemical depression and in alcoholism, and they are close to each other on the same chromosome. Unfortunately, alcohol and sugar are themselves central nervous system depressants (downers). Although they make you feel good temporarily, there is an even deeper plunge into depression afterwards. Exercise, such as jogging, seems to alleviate depression, because it changes brain chemistry.

For reactive depression, people need to keep on feeling the sadness and work the loss through. It is important to acknowledge the depth of the loss and the time needed to get over it.

However, if a person exhibits symptoms of clinical depression, especially of the life-robbing chronic variety, it is essential to seek medical care. Remedies are not the answer to clinical depression. Even if you should succeed in moving the depression out through remedies and other healing tools, there is often a layer of rage underneath that even the most skilled psychotherapists find difficult to handle. If you are a beginning practitioner confronted with a seriously depressed person, you'd do well to refer him or her immediately to a qualified professional.

In general, it's important to ask whether people are on any medication before you start them on flower remedies, but it's crucial if the complaint is depression. My experience with people on strong medication for depression is that antidepressants may sometimes—though not always—wipe out the effects of flower essences. Furthermore, the combination can be unpredictable. The lesser tranquilizers like Valium do not seem to have such a blocking effect. In the following pages, when I say depressed, I will be talking about the garden variety blues.

Bach's Mustard has been described as alleviating the dark depression that descends for no known cause and can lift just as suddenly. To me, this seems to be a biochemically induced mood swing, in that there is no known cause for it.

I have often found Bach's Sweet Chestnut to produce an amazing turnaround in a matter of days for those going through "the dark night of the soul." The classical description says that this remedy is for those who have reached the limit of their endurance, but who are not suicidal.

Similarly, Australian Bush Flower Essences features an essence of the exotic Watarah, which they recommend for this state of mind. I haven't tried it, as I'm sweet on Sweet Chestnut.

Grief—The Modern Taboo

One of the most common sources of reactive depression is grief over the death of a loved one. Grief is one of the emotions our culture most wants us to suppress. Old rituals for mourning, which fostered the grieving process and the healing of the loss, are gone. We still send flowers to funerals, but mourners are expected to return quickly to their usual activities. They don't wear black for a year as they once did, nor are loud lamentations or clothes-rending in vogue. You'd be accused of overreacting if you so much as ripped a sleeve. It is the highest praise to say, "He's taking it very well," when, in fact, the suppression of sorrow should engender some concern.

Mourning that is not dealt with can turn into clinical depression, bitterness, estrangement from the Divine, fear of getting close, or physical illness. It is all too common for the medical establishment—with our complicity—to sedate mourners with tranquilizers so that no one is troubled by their grief. The result of prolonged sedation can be that these feelings are frozen, only to come out strongly with repeated loss. Most men don't like to go to doctors, so they all too often go to bars to medicate their losses. Thus, many drinking problems can be laid at the door of unprocessed grief.

It is important to understand that grief is a process that is not over quickly. When the loved one was close, it could take a year or longer to pick up your life. Often people are numb at the time of the funeral, and then find it increasingly difficult to suppress the sorrow afterwards. You may be all right during the day, only to wake up inconsolable in the middle of the night. Grief ebbs and flows, sometimes seeming to be finished, only to return full force when something reminds you of the loved one. The first full set of meaningful holidays without the departed is often hard. Friends and family members often find it difficult to be supportive over a prolonged period, so it may be useful to join a bereavement group, especially if the loved one did not die peacefully. You may also wish to read the variety of self-help books about the mourning process, such as Eugenia Price's compassionate paperback, *Getting Through the Night* (Ballantine, 1982).

There are a variety of remedies that give courage and strength to work through grief and not get stuck in any of these less desirable manifestations. Bleeding Heart, by FES, is a more general remedy for losses of loved ones, not just through death.

When the grief or sorrow is old, Sturt Desert Pea by Australian Bush Essences is most helpful. Often, it is a cathartic, bringing up the suppressed tears. (Sturt Desert Pea is profiled at the end of the chapter.)

Grief also often contains large admixtures of resentment and guilt, so you might also test for Bach's Willow and Pine—especially if the person is pine-ing away.

Bach's Honeysuckle alleviates the nostalgia and longing for the past that often accompanies grief, so that the individual is able to look forward again and establish a new life.

Grief is not limited to the loss of a loved one. It can come on with a career setback, damage to a part of our self-image, or even the shattering of an ideal. In such situations, you would also want to check out the remedies for grief. However, remedies for despair and discouragement in chapter 9 may be more appropriate. Where self-esteem has been affected by the setback, see chapter 5.

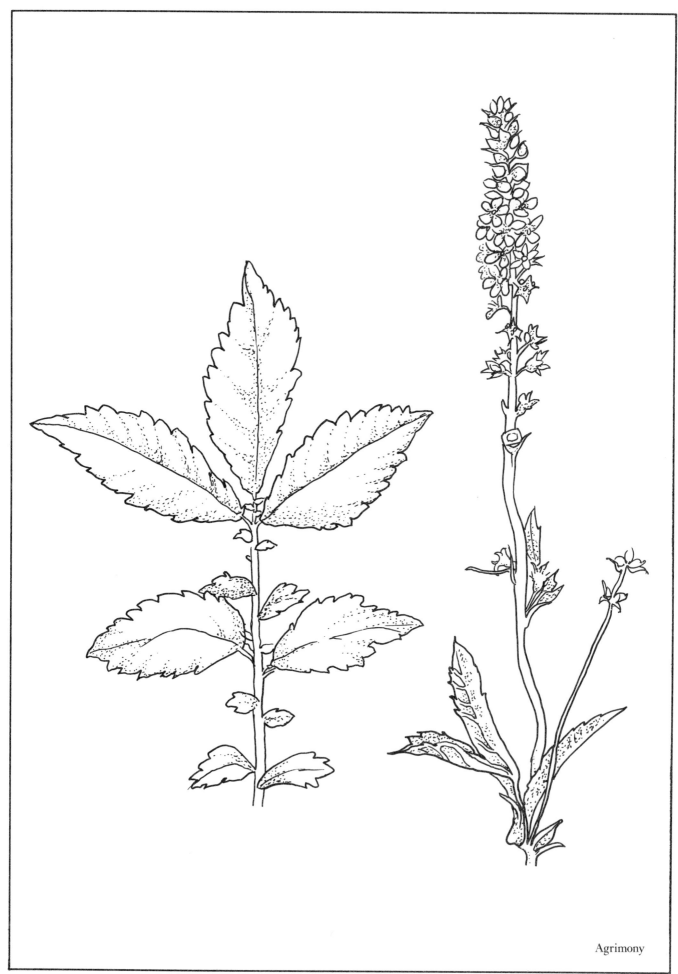

Agrimony

AGRIMONY

Aliases: Latin name *Agrimonia eupatoria*. *Agrimonia* from the original Greek name, *argemōnē*; *eupatoria* for the Greek king Mithridates Eupatōr, who was forever afraid he'd be poisoned and who was said to have discovered that this plant was an antidote to poison. Common names include stickwort, church steeples, and cocklebur.

Companies making the essence: Bach, Healing Herbs, Pegasus.

Essence qualities: For people who are determinedly cheerful and would never complain, but inside are tormented and suffering deeply. Often helpful for the person who drinks or uses other substances to forget the pain and to maintain this façade.

Lore: In the language of flowers, it means "gratitude." It was once believed to have the power to remove curses and send them back to the person who initiated them. People carried agrimony in sachets to protect themselves against evil. It was also burned, with mugwort, for psychic healing and protection. Stuffed into a dream pillow, it was supposedly helpful for people who sleep badly for emotional reasons or because of nagging, persistent thoughts.

What the plant is like: A tall stalk rises above the leaves, with many small yellow flowers on it. Rough seed heads or burrs hang down from the stalk and cling to clothing. It flowers during July and August.

Uses: As an herb, it was used for the liver and gall bladder, for intestinal and urinary irritations, and also as a tonic for muscle tone and for the stomach. Herbalists also claimed that taking daily doses for a year would cure arthritis.

Reflections: Test Agrimony for all with addictive habits, also those in mourning who are "taking it so well." Note the connection between alcoholism and the liver and gall bladder, a primary herbal use of agrimony. Also try the remedy for sleep disturbances, where the person is troubled at night by the feelings not owned during the day, since the herb itself was traditionally used in sleep disturbances.

Affirmations: I PERMIT MYSELF TO SHOW MY REAL
FEELINGS.

MY TRUE SELF IS LOVINGLY SUPPORTED
BY THOSE AROUND ME.

I NOW RELEASE THE PAIN I AM HOLDING.

Astrological correlations: According to Culpeper, agrimony is connected with Jupiter and Cancer. The remedy seems likely for those with fire signs rising (Aries, Leo, or Sagittarius), but who are more watery by nature, having the Sun or Moon in the water signs Cancer, Scorpio, or Pisces.

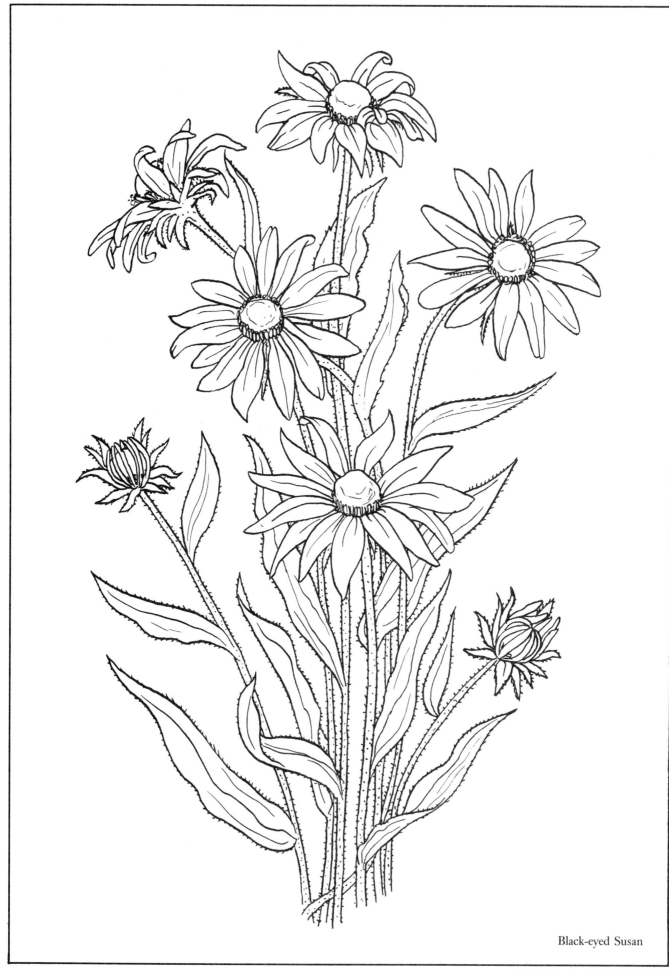

Black-eyed Susan

BLACK-EYED SUSAN

Aliases: Latin name *Rudbeckia hirta*. *Hirta* means hairy; *Rudbeckia* for botanist Olaf Rudbeck. Also commonly called rudbeckia.

Companies making the essence: FES, Pegasus.

Essence qualities: The FES description says that in the counseling process, it helps release resistance to and avoidance of looking at emotions. Brings penetrating insight into deep emotions and the darker side of the soul. Helps to raise low self-esteem.

Lore: In the language of flowers, it meant justice. State flower of Maryland.

What the plant is like: A smaller member of the sunflower and coneflower family, only 1′ to 3′ (30 cm to 1 m) tall with blooms 2″ to 3″ (5 cm to 7 cm) across. It shares the bright golden petals and the black disk in the center, although the disk is often dome-shaped. Some species also have a reddish brown coloration of the petals, near the disk. Long-flowering, it blooms from June to October. It grows in sunny areas, but is a hardy plant and not at all fussy about growing conditions.

Uses: Native Americans drank a tea of the roots as a cold medicine. FES says that, herbally, it was used to treat boils, and notes that the dark, protruding center resembles a boil.

Reflections: This essence seems likely to help people accept and embrace their shadow, as represented by the blackness at the center of the flower. Since the plant is related to the sunflower, it is not surprising that, like Sunflower essence, Black-eyed Susan has been helpful in raising self-esteem. Here the increased self-esteem would be due to its usefulness in accepting rather than avoiding unacceptable emotions and the shadow side of the self.

Affirmations: I FACE MY FEELINGS FEARLESSLY AND ACCEPT THEM.

I CONFRONT MY SHADOW AND BRING IT LOVINGLY TO THE LIGHT.

I RELEASE ALL OBSTACLES TO ACCEPTING THE HELP I NEED.

Astrological correlations: People who need Black-eyed Susan would have Neptune aspects to the Moon in their birth charts or Moon in Pisces. It would also help during transits by Pluto to the Moon or Neptune. However, since there is some association with the Sun as well, it may be useful for those born at the Full Moon, first or third quarters, who have a hard time reconciling their feelings with their self-concept.

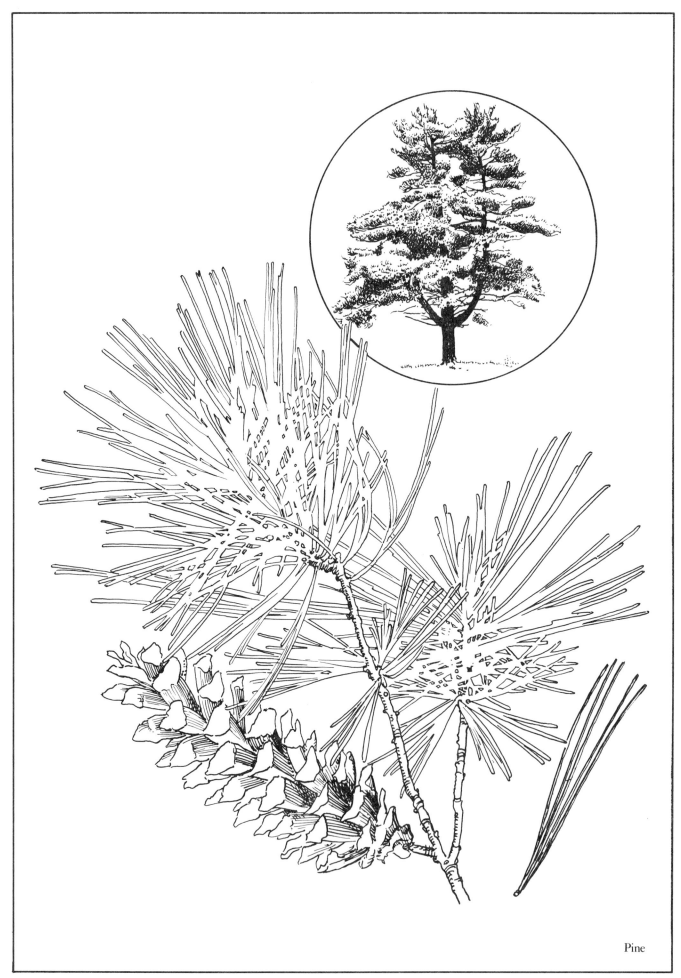

Pine

PINE

Aliases: Latin name *Pinus sylvestris*. The word *pinus* means pine tree. *Sylvestris* refers to forest.

Companies making the essence: Bach, FES, Healing Herbs, Pegasus.

Essence qualities: It works against guilt, self-reproach, blaming self for the mistakes of others.

Lore: Pine was sacred to Poseidon, so in ancient Greece sailors would use the pitch in their boats to be safe on the waters. Pine was sacred to the Druids, who carried the cones as fertility symbols. The Druids threw the needles on the floor to cleanse negativity and burned them to reverse spells. However, to the early Christians, a pine cone cut length-wise resembled a hand. Thus, it reminded them of Jesus' hand, which he used to bless the pine because it sheltered his mother when she was in flight from Herod. In Japan, it was customary to place a pine branch over the door of the house to ensure continual joy, for the leaves are evergreen. In the Japanese flower calendar, it was the flower of the month for January. In the language of flowers, it meant "pity."

What the plant is like: An evergreen tree, with long needles, and cones for seeds. Its height varies with age and specific variety, from 3′ (1 m) to 50′ (15 m) or more.

Uses: Boiled in vinegar, pine needles were an old-time remedy for tooth-ache. Also, the unripe cones were soaked in water, and the water was then used as a wrinkle remedy. It was also recommended as a relaxing and healthful bath. Thought to relieve arthritis, the needles and buds were boiled until the water was very aromatic, then the water was added to the bath. Inhaled, pine made a cold remedy. The needles were burned during the winter months to purify the house. The resin was used in incense, as it was said to clear negative energy from a space. Because of the healthful qualities of the smell, sanitariums were often located in pine forests.

Reflections: Just as pine is a cleanser and purifier on the physical level, so can Pine essence be on a spiritual and emotional level.

Affirmations: I LET GO OF GUILT THAT DOESN'T BELONG TO ME.

I TAKE RESPONSIBILITY FOR MY MISDEEDS AND LEARN FROM THEM.

I ACCEPT MY SHORTCOMINGS AS HUMAN AND FORGIVE MYSELF.

WHERE POSSIBLE, I MAKE AMENDS TO THOSE I HARMED.

Astrological correlations: People with a strong Neptune and/or Pluto are often guilt-ridden, as are those with strong Virgo influences.

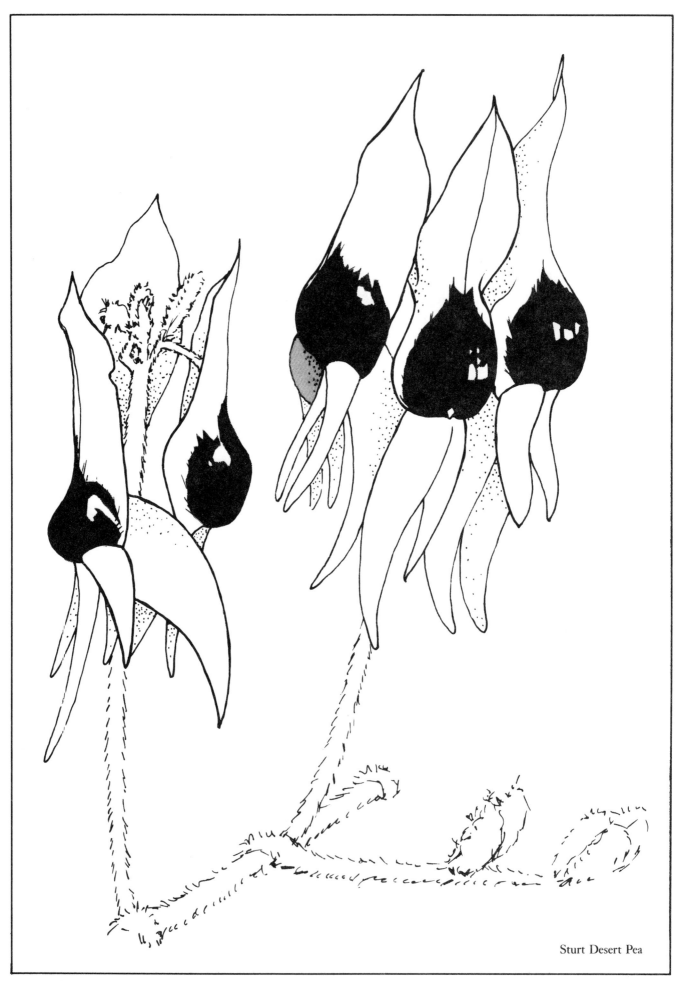

Sturt Desert Pea

STURT DESERT PEA

Aliases: Latin name *Clianthus formosus*. *Clianthus* from the Greek *kleos*, meaning glory, and *anthos*, meaning flower; *formosus* meaning beautiful or well formed. Named for the Australian explorer Charles Sturt who first described this flower, it is listed as Sturt's Desert Pea in botanical reference books.

Companies making the essence: Australian Bush Flower Essences.

Essence qualities: In his book *Australian Bush Flower Essences*, Ian White describes this essence as being a powerful one for processing and releasing old sorrows, even those from past lives.[3]

Lore: Floral emblem of South Australia. To the Aboriginals, as portrayed in their legends, the flower symbolized blood, loss, and grief.

What the plant is like: The pea pod-shaped annual flowers are striking—bright red with a glossy, black knob like a pea at the center. The long, narrow flowers are from about 1″ to 4″ (2 cm to 10 cm) in length, grow low to the ground, and hang from short stems in clusters of four or five. They bloom in sandy, arid areas throughout Australia in the tropical fall, winter, and spring, especially after heavy rains. The seeds—which are legumes like garden peas—are in pods 2″ to 2½″ (5 cm to 6 cm) long, but they are hard to germinate and may not sprout until after a fire or being boiled. Ian White notes that they have been known to sprout after as much as 40 years, like old sorrows.

Uses: No herbal properties noted. The Australian Bush Essences have a number of cases on record of the essence having a powerful effect on physical illnesses such as lung disease or arthritis, as the individual experienced and released the old grief.

Reflections: The black-and-red flower seems to me to illustrate principles about grief, with the black representing mourning and the red portraying the anger that so often surrounds it. Red also represents life force and vitality, so the black knob in the center shows that holding grief in can deaden vitality, whereas experiencing the grief and the accompanying anger can bring renewed strength and energy.

Affirmations: I GIVE MYSELF PERMISSION TO RELEASE MY SADNESS.

I ALLOW MYSELF TO EXPERIENCE ALL MY FEELINGS.

I AM FREE OF MY SORROW ABOUT _____.

Astrological correlations: The person with Pluto strong in the birth chart—especially in the first or fourth house or aspecting the Moon—has often experienced early and repeated grief, so might well benefit from a course of Sturt Desert Pea. The person who has had a number of Pluto transits over the past several years should also be tested for it.

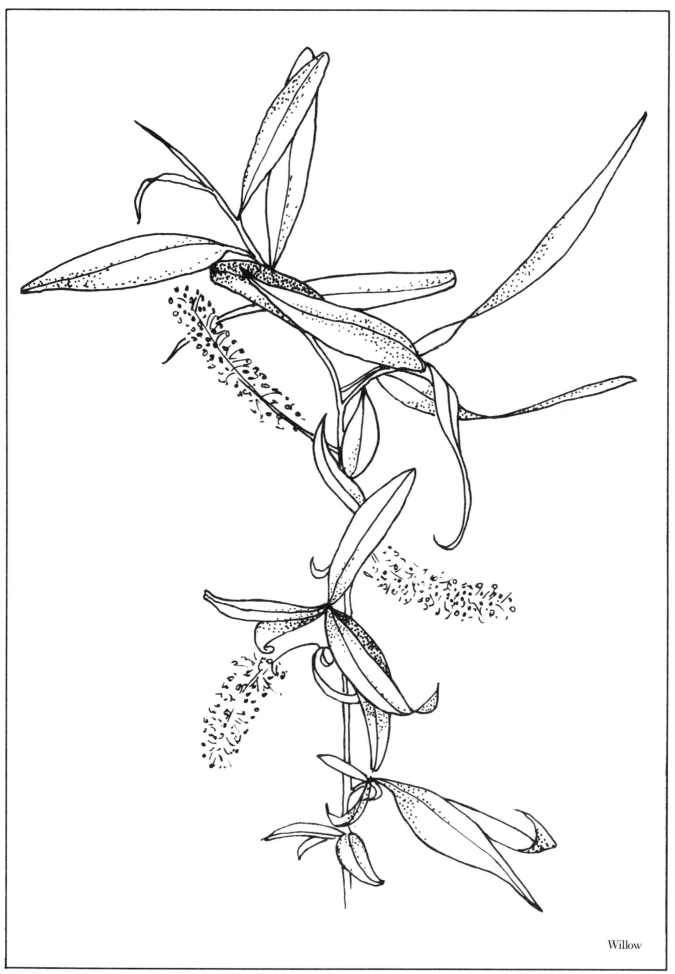

Willow

WILLOW

Aliases: Latin name *Salix vitellina*. *Salix* probably derived from two Celtic words, *sal* and *lis*, meaning near water; *vitellina* meant golden-haired. Common names included osier, saille, and witches' aspirin.

Companies making the essence: Alaskan Flower Essence Project, Bach, Healing Herbs, Pegasus.

Essence qualities: For resentments and grudges, but more especially for embittered individuals or injustice collectors, who brood and think of themselves as victims, begrudging the happiness of others. Such habits drive people away, so these individuals become increasingly isolated.

Lore: For centuries, the willow has been associated with both death and immortality. The Chinese saw it as a symbol of immortality, because you can grow a new tree from the smallest branch. In Greek and Roman mythology, the willow is sacred to Circe, Hecate, and Persephone, all death aspects of the Mother Goddess. It became a symbol of mourning—especially the weeping willow. Its symbolic meaning is forsaken love. Druid tree sign for April 16 to May 13; flower of the month for November in the Japanese flower calendar; birthday flower for May 22.

What the plant is like: This tall tree is often found growing on river banks because the roots bind the soil. The flowers are long yellow or green pendants called catkins.

Uses: Widely used as a sedative by herbalists, the bark was, until the early 1900s, the only source of salicylic acid, an ingredient in aspirin. Salicin, extracted from the bark, was substituted for quinine against malaria. Used for eye drops, as an astringent, and as a detergent.

Reflections: Useful for the bereaved, who are often unconsciously enraged about their loss. The threat of loss of love often leads people to avoid conflict, but suppressed anger turns into resentment. Our deepest resentments are often toward those we once loved.

Affirmations: I WILLINGLY RELEASE THE HABIT OF RESENTMENT.

SO THAT I MAY BE WHOLE, I LET GO OF MY RESENTMENT TOWARD (NAME).

I TAKE RESPONSIBILITY FOR MY OWN MISFORTUNES.

Astrological correlations: For people who have a strong Pluto or Scorpio component in their birth charts, especially after Pluto squares Pluto (ages 40 to 43).

Flower Remedies—A Way to Feel Differently

With these essences, you have a powerful new tool for dealing with emotions. Using them takes a certain amount of work and courage. They don't make the feelings go away—wouldn't it be grand if they did! What they do instead is help you move through them more quickly, transmuting them so that you don't get stuck in them. As you take them, your Higher Self, rather than your lower self or your ego, becomes engaged in the process. Thus, you gain self-understanding and learn how to deal with upsetting situations more effectively. They also help clear out the backlog of emotions accumulated in a lifetime of avoidance. Although they cannot replace therapy when that is needed, they are an excellent adjunct to it, often speeding the process.

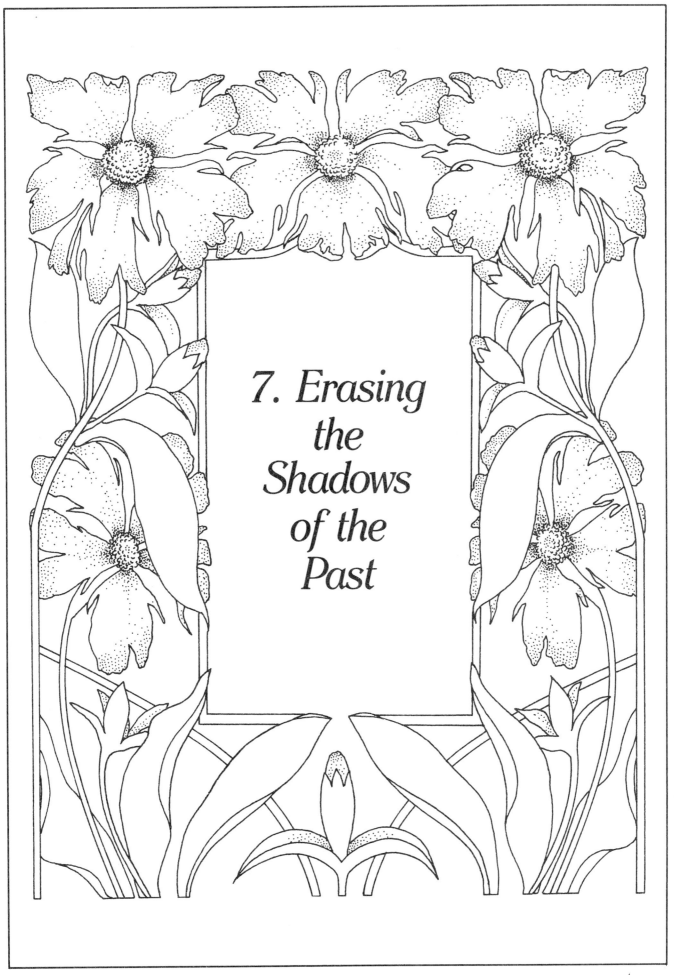

7. Erasing the Shadows of the Past

In this chapter, we will discuss difficult topics like incest, child abuse, rape, and other victim experiences, and the effects of growing up in a seriously dysfunctional family. When past events have been damaging, they tend to leave residues that affect present functioning. We'll find ways to recognize the shadows of the past, and we'll discuss remedies and other tools to help release them.

If you have had difficult experiences such as these, this material may guide your own healing. If you haven't, you may want to skip over it until you have occasion to use the information for someone else. However, if you are a practitioner, this chapter will be particularly useful.

What is the definition of a practitioner? The first time you gave a remedy to someone other than yourself—your child, or even your dog—you became an apprentice practitioner. Maybe you don't feel ready to become one, but that is what the more advanced material in this chapter and others will prepare you for.

Some Explanations to Practitioners

Much of the information given here is not just about flower remedies but about syndromes related to such damaging histories and about strategies of treatment. It is based on my own extensive experience and that of others who work with such clients. This information is included because histories like these leave serious residues and because we are seeing more and more of them. As the recovery movement continues to grow, survivors become increasingly vocal about their experiences and are ready to heal themselves and be free. It is important for you to recognize the symptoms and to be prepared with more than flower remedies should these people come to you. The essences can play an important part, and there are some of special relevance to these issues, but they cannot do it alone.

More people than you'd think have had such experiences. The statistics are that one woman in three has suffered from sexual abuse; at least 10 percent of all children have been physically abused; close to one woman in three has been battered by her mate; and at least one person in four has been strongly affected by his or her relationship with an addict.

There is a tendency among a certain kind of New Age disciple simply to declare the past irrelevant. They want to believe that having taken a workshop or two, pounded a few pillows, said some affirmations, and discovered the terrible things you did in your past lives, you should now be healed. If you are not, these so-called metaphysicians are likely to tell you smugly that you chose the experience for some reason.

Would that it were so simple. Healing from a serious wounding or dysfunctional family is long and arduous. It requires great courage on the part of the survivor and great compassion on the part of the practitioner. If you have survived a background like this, you will need to talk about the experience over and over, venting the feelings. You may have to come back to the same issue time and again, as healing proceeds on deeper and deeper levels. We may be talking about a year or two here, not just a few sessions. Insight does not end the process—it only begins it.

Ways the essences can contribute are to help people to face the associated emotions with courage, release them more quickly and completely, and restore themselves at points of weariness along the way. We discussed Black-eyed Susan, Fuchsia, and Scarlet Monkeyflower earlier for facing and integrating emotions, and these are especially helpful when dealing with the feelings that come up in recovery.

Borage gives courage in adversity.

Oak is a solace to those who have had a long, hard struggle.

Desert Alchemy describes one effect of Aloe Vera as a surrendering to the healing process with a sense of joy and being supported from within.

Desert Alchemy also recommends Bisbee Beehive Cactus, profiled at the end of this chapter, for healing serious childhood wounds, particularly sexual abuse. They say it helps penetrate to the core of an issue and heal at a cellular level.

The Need for a Holistic Approach

It is important to stress once more that essences alone are not enough when the person has been a victim of abuse or violence. In working with many such people over the years, I find a combination of treatments is required for wholeness—not only individual psychotherapy and essences but bodywork, energy work, and groups. Otherwise, clients may have insights galore, but painful patterns related to those events do not change. Insight without change only reinforces their feelings of helplessness and hopelessness.

Where the violation has been physical, gentler forms of bodywork like massage are needed. Gentle handling conveys the message that it is safe to release the tension. The body remains on guard after any serious shock, so there is a residue of tension and stress.

Star of Bethlehem is an invaluable remedy for old shocks and traumas. The body has an amazing capacity to remember, in vivid detail, everything that ever happened to it. It is as conscious as the mind. If you earnestly and consistently convey a desire to communicate, you will be surprised what your body tells you.

It also holds intense *feelings* about what happened, which only body- and energy work can release. Such stored feelings can act as a block against intimacy, no matter how much the mind and heart might desire closeness. If the person fears being touched, try the essences in chapter 4, particularly Dandelion and Flannel Flower.

The aura also needs clearing so the person does not continue to attract the same damaging types of people or experiences. We attract people and are attracted through the intermingling of energy bodies, as much as by physical appearance. This interaction is mostly outside our awareness, but we may allude to it in statements like "I don't know, I just didn't like his energy."

Albeit unconsciously, the former victim is often *energetically recognized* by potential victimizers and singled out as ripe for further abuse. Strong, undischarged emotions also create blockages in the chakras, especially the heart, which we will be working with in chapter 8. So long as fear, guilt, sorrow, or anger are held in the aura, they present a barrier to healthy energy exchange with others. Some of the remedies we have already discussed, such as Pine for guilt and Rock Rose for fear, can help clear the energy field.

Fortunately, we live in an era when all these secrets are coming into the open and when there are a variety of twelve-step groups, therapy groups, crime victim programs, and even social action groups for these purposes. Many who need them, however, have difficulty joining a group, out of the trust and shame issues that so often result from violation. If so, essences described in the section on groups in chapter 4 will help remove that barrier, especially Mariposa Lily and Violet.

A good self-help book can start the process of recovery, even when survivors are not ready or able to seek help more formally. They can read it in privacy, not having to deal with anyone else as their barriers come down. The stories in the books let them know that they are not alone. They also learn the effects such experiences have on adult functioning. A good combination to take while reading would be Desert Alchemy's Releasing Judgment and Denial.

It is important for the practitioner to be able to recommend some currently available self-help books. Visit self-help sections of local bookstores or the public library. Get catalogs from Hazelden, Compcare, or Health Communication, all major and respected sources of recovery literature.

It might strengthen your understanding of dysfunctional family background to read these books yourself. Calendula by FES would help increase the ability to listen or read receptively.

Belonging to Alcoholic or Dysfunctional Families

Statistics show that one person in four has been deeply affected by a relationship with an alcoholic. Therefore, if you are a practitioner, 25 percent or more of the people who come to you as clients are family members, lovers, or close friends of alcoholics. If you aren't finding this to be true of your clients, maybe they're not telling you this family secret out of shame or they don't think you need to know.[1]

It isn't simply a case of being secretive. One major trait of families of alcoholics or addicts is that everyone, beginning with the alcoholic, tends to deny the addiction. This protects the addict in the habit and protects the family from the pain and shame of seeing how destructive a problem it is. Denial means that they either don't recognize that an addiction exists or that they're addicted to the addict. Many see the addiction and yet deny the extent of the damage. Adult children of alcoholics (ACAs) say things like "Yes, my dad drank, but he stopped when I was sixteen, and it doesn't have any bearing on my life today." As we'll see later, the residuals are considerable, especially in the ways these people relate and work.

The Desert Alchemy combination mentioned earlier, Releasing Denial and Judgment, would also be useful for ACAs.

Remedies for shame, such as Bach's Crab Apple and Desert Alchemy's Foothills Paloverde, may also be a solace.

In his important and readable book *A Primer for Adult Children of Alcoholics*, psychiatrist Timmen

Cermak discusses the major characteristics of ACAs. Although not every ACA has all of them, these are common. They are fearful and especially fear their feelings (Scarlet Monkeyflower or Fuchsia), losing control (Vine), conflict, authority figures, and angry people. Although they're fiercely self-critical and suffer from low self-esteem, they're frightened of criticism from others, so they constantly seek approval (Cymbidium). ACAs feel guilty standing up for themselves (Pine) and so take on too much responsibility. They have a special area of difficulty in intimate relationships. Because they're afraid of being abandoned, they'll do almost anything to hold on to relationships, which are often with addictive personalities or other unavailable people. They confuse love and pity, often attaching themselves to others who are victims or whom they can rescue. They may also place themselves repeatedly in the victim role (Centaury).[2]

Although we will focus on alcoholic families in this discussion, other addictions and serious family dysfunctions can also take their toll. Unhappy experiences such as having a schizophrenic or chronically depressed parent, a parent or sibling who dies early, or a severely abusive sibling can all leave residues of pain that may need to be healed. If you came from a nightmare background, you may strongly identify with the characteristics of ACAs listed earlier and may find the ACA groups healing as well. Two main effects of growing up in an alcoholic or dysfunctional home relate to love and career. To find remedies for the effects on relationships of growing up in a dysfunctional family, see the section on codependency in chapter 8; for the effects on career, see chapter 9.

Long-Range Effects of Sexual Abuse

The following list of traits of incest survivors circulated at various twelve-step meetings was compiled by E. Sue Blume, CSW, a Long Island psychotherapist.[3] The survivor may exhibit many of these traits: fear of being alone, especially in the dark; nightmares, especially of pursuit; alienation from the body and not heeding its signals; eating disorders and other addictions; the need to feel invisible; depression; and low self-esteem. They

also suffer from shame and guilt, feeling different, compulsive behaviors, trust issues, taking excessive risks or being afraid to take any at all. Other tendencies include the pattern of being a victim, power and control issues, fear of anger or being angry all the time.

In addition, there are relationships in which true intimacy cannot occur, sexual dysfunctions or sexual compulsions, swallowing or gagging sensitivity, and wearing excessive or baggy clothing, even in summer. Some of these difficulties can be attributed to other causes, but if a number of them are present, you might suspect abuse of some kind.

Although boys suffer from molestation and sexual abuse more often than you imagine, it is even harder for them to accept or talk about. They worry that it impugns their manhood or that someone might think they were gay. Only now that the incest recovery movement has endured for several years are men beginning to speak up.

Men with this history might profit from Flannel Flower by Australian Bush Flower Essences, as well as the essences discussed below.

Sexual abuse or sexual assault has serious effects on the energy body, which also needs to be healed for the person to be whole. The sexual chakra is located below the navel in women and in the area of the testicles in men. Although younger children can have sexual feelings, it is normal for this chakra to begin opening in earnest in the early to middle teens. It may open too early when a child is molested, the victim of incest, or even repeatedly subjected to exposure to activities of a promiscuous or oversexed parent. When the chakra is opened early and too much energy diverted to it, the development of other chakras is distorted.

Remedies that relieve the effects of molestation on the energy body are Bisbee Beehive Cactus, by Desert Alchemy, Fringed Violet, by the Australian Bush Flower Essences, and Macrozamia, by Living Essences.

In the chapter on self-esteem, we talked about the normal development of the chakra system and the crucial role of the solar plexus in the younger child. The solar plexus is located directly above the sexual chakra, so there is an easy spillover effect. Given a low self-concept, children of alcoholics are vulnerable to sexual abuse or to using sex to bolster self-worth.

The practitioner should test for Crab Apple. In addition to clearing the sexual chakra, solar plexus and self-esteem work may be needed.

There may also be effects on current sexual functioning, which can best be addressed after the emotional layers are cleared out. Some are left fearful of sexuality and find ways to keep it out of their lives. Hibiscus and Sticky Monkeyflower by FES can help with the fear of intimacy.

Billy Goat Plum, by Australian Bush Essences, can help those who are repelled by sex and by their own sex organs.

Sexual anxiety can be masked by other symptoms. Addiction is a common response, used to numb fear of sexual connection. Some become workaholics who can't make time in their busy lives for sexuality. Others either have relationships with unavailable people who make few demands or avoid relationships altogether. Each of these problems can have other origins, often multiple causes.

Alternately, the child who is prematurely exposed to sexuality can grow up to be sexually compulsive. This is because the sexual chakra is overdeveloped, fed energy at the expense of other chakras. Sexuality then serves many other purposes besides the physical. For example, it serves to control others or to keep them at a distance, to get revenge on parents, or to appease the desperate loneliness that the betrayal and the shameful secret leaves in its wake. Where control issues dominate relationships, test for Bach's Vine.

In our era, deadly sexually transmitted diseases make this group vulnerable and thus in urgent need of healing. Therapy, the essences, body- and energy work will change that pattern. Try Bach's Cherry Plum, which is often useful in changing self-destructive habits.

What If You Don't Remember?

What if you score high on the lists of traits of incest survivors or adult children of alcoholics, but don't remember anything of the sort? Sometimes I have encountered people who were seriously ill during long periods of early childhood and had difficult medical treatments that were physically invasive. As adults, they have some ACA or incest-survivor symptoms. Grandchildren of alcoholics can have every trait on the ACA list, even when the parents are teetotalers. The grandparents pass the syndrome on to the parents, who pass it on to the children—a kind of emotional legacy of learned behaviors.

More often, there is a kind of amnesia about the abuse. Many victims of violation in infancy have no memory of the events because they did not possess the language to comprehend what happened. A more complete childhood amnesia—for instance, those who have little or no memory of certain years of their childhood—usually means prolonged and serious disturbance in the home and most likely some kind of abuse.

Others remember parts of childhood but in an oddly distanced way, as though it all happened to someone else. There are often great gaps in memory and alienation from the body.

FES's Golden Eardrops, for clearing sadness related to an unhappy childhood, may be useful.

I advise caution in dealing with childhood amnesia. Even though the memories are not conscious, the mind is strongly protecting the individual by blanking out what happened. There is no point in pushing or in resorting to hypnosis. When the Higher Self knows the person is strong enough, memories will begin to trickle through, perhaps in dreams. If you are the individual, you can reassure the Higher Self of your readiness by communicating willingness to go through the emotions that come up. You can surround yourself with healers and other support systems. Often, bodywork will bring up memories. Writing stories about childhood, painting, or drawing may release memories. However, if nothing emerges, let it be. Your Higher Self will know the right time. Even if you never remember, try the remedies given later for releasing the damage of abuse, and they will help.

The Process of Healing from Trauma

Most survivors of serious wounding—from childhood abuse to criminal assault as an adult—function in denial until they feel able to handle the healing process. They may remember the ordeal and even acknowledge that it affected them, yet they remain emotionally detached. They may even believe they've gotten over it. However, most of the time they haven't; they just encapsulated it. The event was so damaging, they couldn't have done anything else.

When the trauma is a physical one, let's say a serious accident, ongoing health care and bodywork can be augmented by several remedies. FES's Arnica restores breaks in life force after shock and injury. It helps maintain connection with one's Higher Self, especially when there is disassociation from the body.

Aloe Vera, discussed on page 53, also helps restore the life force.

Black Cohosh, recommended earlier for emotional trauma, is said by Matt Wood to be specifically helpful in whiplash injuries.

Bach's Star of Bethlehem, profiled at the end of the chapter, is an extremely important remedy for releasing physical shocks and old traumas. It does not seem to matter how long ago the injury took place, this remedy releases deeply held tension from the energy body. The person who needs Star of Bethlehem is often numb, subdued, and shut down to new experience.

Remedies for the Residues of a Difficult Childhood

In addition to therapy, support groups, and bodywork, there are remedies to facilitate the healing process. A crucial one is FES's Golden Eardrops,

which is said to help a person contact and release painful feelings from an unhappy childhood, especially if it was too traumatic to acknowledge at the time. In releasing unhappy memories, the individual may release repressed tears. This pattern of being healed through crying has resulted in this essence being nicknamed "Golden Teardrops." Where there has been loss of a parent because of death or desertion, the remedies for grief given in chapter 6 may also be important.

The *Flower Essence Repertory* recommends Yerba Santa for gentle release of held-in trauma from childhood.[4]

FES's Saguaro, profiled later, helps where there was a problem with the father, especially with regard to his authority. Sunflower can also be helpful where the relationship with the father was damaging to the self-esteem.

Australian Bush Flower Essences recommends Red Helmet for those who had a difficult relationship with their father and who wind up with authority problems. (It is also recommended for men who are adjusting to fatherhood.)

We discussed Mariposa Lily, by FES, as a remedy for alienation and feeling separate and unloved. It increases one's receptivity to human love. FES recommends it for all childhood traumas, but especially where the mother-child bond was not good or was interrupted.

Lady's Mantle, by Harebell, is for those who wish to be in touch with the feminine aspects of the Divine. Therefore, it should help those who are alienated from women and their own feminine side because of negative experiences with the mother or other women in authority.

Test, too, for Desert Alchemy's Milky Nipple Cactus, where there are thorny mother issues.

Remedies to Help Heal Emotional Traumas

Bach's Star of Bethlehem, mentioned for physical traumas, is perhaps the single most crucial remedy for anyone who has suffered from abuse, rape, or assault. No matter how long ago the violation occurred, the energy body is still contracted, fearful of a new violation. Star of Bethlehem, which may be needed for several months in serious cases, helps the energy body relax and reenergize.

I am also having good results by adding Fringed Violet, by Australian Bush Essences. Founder Ian White says that it treats damage to the aura where there has been shock, grief, or physical trauma, such as sexual abuse or assault—either recent or long ago. It results in reintegration of the physical and etheric bodies. It is crucial where the person is still fearful of physical contact.

FES's Manzanita can alleviate deep-seated aversion to being in the physical body because of such experiences.

Perelandra, whose remedies are mostly made from garden vegetables, features two that can be helpful to the person who has been or is being abused.

Their Broccoli alleviates the sense of powerlessness under threat or stress because of closing down for self-protection. It enables the person to function and confront the threat.

Their Comfrey is described as repairing higher-vibration soul damage resulting from trauma in this or other lifetimes. Use in combination with other essences more directly related to the cause of the damage. I give Comfrey now to almost all adult children of dysfunctional families and victims of abuse. This important herb and flower essence, with its long healing history, is profiled at the end of the chapter.

FES's Black Cohosh is an indispensable healer for those who have been powerless—and especially

 107

those who continue to be powerless in the present. I test it for all clients who have been in or are currently in abusive situations. In *Seven Herbs*, Matthew Wood devotes an entire chapter to Black Cohosh, drawing a brilliant portrait of the psychological type who needs it. He says the person tends to be the dark, intense, even brooding type who gets enmeshed in abusive and exploitative relationships and has difficulty getting out. They hesitate to discuss their history with anyone, as they feel no one will believe how bad it was.[5]

Dr. Bach described Centaury as being for weakness of will and those who let themselves be exploited or imposed on by others. What Bach didn't seem to elicit from his patients in the 1930s was whether any of them were victims of abuse or sexual assault. The person who has once been victimized, especially as a young child, often takes on a victim posture and is subjected to repeated victimization. Even when relationships are not overtly abusive, the person may be exploited and taken advantage of. Thus, I test Centaury also for all who have been victims. (It is profiled at the end of the chapter.)

One practitioner who had been severely emotionally abused as a child was frequently taken advantage of by clients. She prided herself on being "a good sport" about missed appointments, long-unpaid bills, repeated bounced checks, clients coming late, and overlong sessions. Although often irritated by such behavior, she was unable to confront offending clients. After only a week of Centaury, she began to stand up for herself and set limits. The work she did was actually better

afterwards, she came to see, because many of her clients had boundary issues too.

Another pattern for those who had difficult childhoods can be helped by the Australian Bush Essences' Southern Cross. It is specifically for bitter, complaining people, and martyrs with poverty consciousness. Founder Ian White says that taking Southern Cross helps them understand that in adulthood they create the situations that happen to them, so that they are able to take responsibility and regain a sense of personal power.

As mentioned earlier, in the healing process there are successive stages of intense feelings about the damaging events. Remedies for each emotion given in chapter 6 will help these stages pass more quickly, with more complete release of the residues.

Special mention is due Holly, for hatred and the desire for revenge; Vervain, for people who are incensed at injustices; and Willow, for bitterness and resentment.

The various remedies for grief should also be considered, because grief over the loss of wholeness and the destruction of the important relationship involved is an important stage.

Sturt Desert Pea, for releasing old grief and sorrow, has been particularly helpful at this time.

A Case History

This chapter has been the most difficult to find suitable case histories for, even though people like these just mentioned have long made up part of my practice. There are several reasons for this lack. One is out of respect for my clients' privacy, because I do not divulge personal details of their stories. Confidentiality is an absolute requirement for this work. The secrets people share with you must be respected and held in absolute trust. It is all the more vital in a book like this. It is one thing

to share your secrets with a practitioner, one on one. It is another thing altogether to read about yourself in a book, even when you gave the practitioner permission to put it there. No one wants to be regarded as a case. I offer my thanks to the clients who gave me permission to print their stories.

Another difficulty is that flower essence work with those who have traumatic histories tends to be a very long process, with many of the essences repeated at different points in time. There is no neat beginning and end. It is difficult to decipher what effects the remedies had, as opposed to the other kinds of work the client is simultaneously involved in. (I insist on a holistic approach, with a variety of resources.)

One writer to whom I gave essences came from a minority background of severe hardship and many losses, with drug addiction in the family and an alcohol problem he himself had successfully put down for a number of years. He got a contract to write a book for children who have addiction in the family—a poignant, yet healing and rewarding topic for him. The project was stalled many times: writing about the past brought up feelings that were difficult to deal with. At one point when it was almost finished but stalled again, he asked for some remedies to help him get through it.

I gave him FES's Golden Eardrops (twice), for gaining a new perspective on unhappy childhood memories, their Scarlet Monkeyflower, for integrating strong emotions, and Petite Fleur's Orchid, for making peace with the past. These remedies brought up some sorrow, yet he found himself thinking and feeling differently. The work began to move forward again.

As so often happens, another layer came to the surface. Always a feisty individual, he found he was now angry at the ignorance and bigotry of people from more privileged backgrounds. This anger was bursting out in situations he found inappropriate and even potentially professionally damaging.

For this, I twice mixed Vervain, for those who are incensed at injustices, Scarlet Monkeyflower, for integrating strong emotions, and Fireweed, for releasing old angers. The anger began to pass and he found he was handling people differently—no less self-assertive, but cooler and more tactfully.

When the final draft of the book was due and he was stuck again, I mixed him a new combination containing several of the former remedies as well as Madia, for follow-through and concentration, Iris, for creativity, and Comfrey, for healing soul damage.

Remedies for Letting Go of the Past

There are useful remedies for letting go of the past. Orchid, by Petite Fleur, allows one to make peace with it.

The Alaskan Flower Essence Project makes three remedies I find important in completing the healing.

Sitka Burnet helps to heal the past and reach completion.

Their Mountain Wormwood is a very important remedy for healing old wounds and releasing unforgiven areas in our relationships with others and with the self. Here, it is important not to rush to a superficial and phony forgiveness that essentially short-circuits the healing process. You must work through all the feelings about the abuse or betrayal before you can reach any real point of forgiveness. Many workers in the field of incest and abuse recovery state that forgiveness is not a goal, but sometimes is an end product of the work.

Finally, River Beauty helps a person in starting over after a devastating experience, regeneration, and seeing adverse circumstances as potential for cleansing and growth.

Two essences are helpful in releasing a long, hard struggle. Bach's Oak is an important restorative for those who have long contended with hardship.

Sunshine Wattle, by Australian Bush Remedies, presents a different outlook on life, for those who've had a difficult time in the past and who are stuck there, bringing those negative experiences into the present.

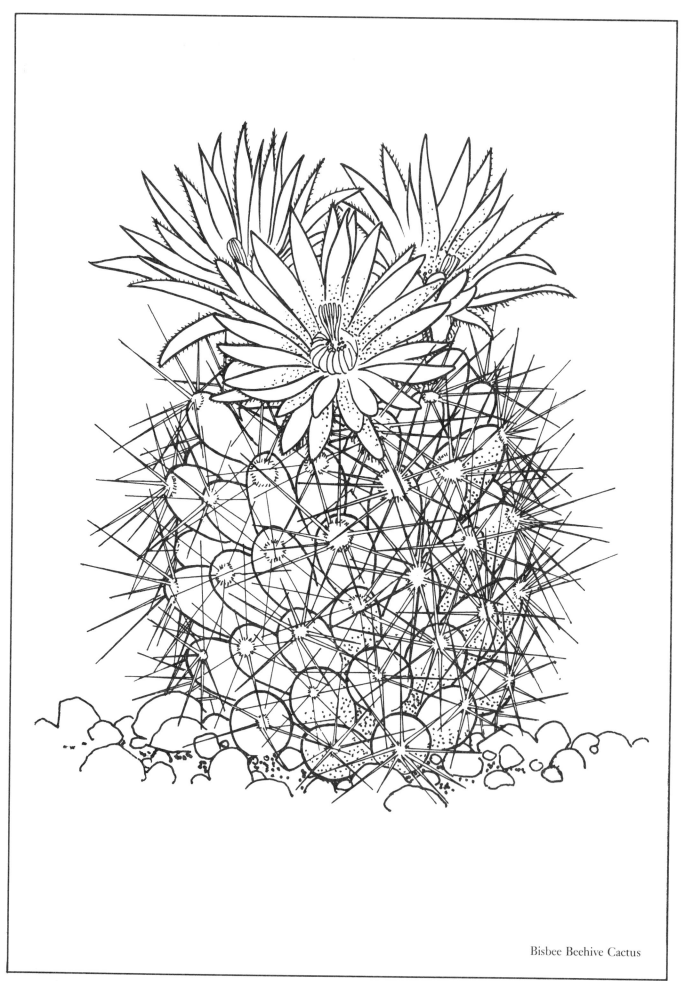

Bisbee Beehive Cactus

BISBEE BEEHIVE CACTUS

Aliases: Latin name *Coryphantha vivipara*. *Coryphanta* means top flower. *Vivipara* means germinating or sprouting while still attached.

Company making the essence: Desert Alchemy.

Essence qualities: Desert Alchemy's catalog says that this essence goes to the core of an issue and allows you to feel grace and healing energy on a cellular level. They particularly recommend it for healing sexual abuse.

Lore: None found.

What the plant is like: This small ball-shaped or columnar cactus is often kept as a houseplant. It can grow in groups or mounds as high as 1½′ (0.45 m). It is hardy and can resist frost, but requires some shade. It is covered with circles of long spines, radiating out from the center. In summer, there are beautiful, delicately colored pink flowers.

Uses: Ornamental.

Reflections: The spines that radiate out from the center of a circle of spines are reminiscent of the Sun, which is *the* center. They also suggest the remedy's property of going to the core of an issue.

Affirmations: I FIND THE DEEPER MEANINGS OF MY PROBLEM.

HEALING PROCEEDS TO THE DEEPEST LEVEL OF MY BEING.

IT WILL BE ALL RIGHT.

GRACE UNFOLDS WITHIN ME.

Astrological correlations: This remedy could be used during Pluto transits, because the most positive use of Pluto is healing and transformation of old wounds. People who have Pluto in the first house of their birth chart, on the Midheaven, or conjunct Mars may particularly need Bisbee Beehive Cactus.

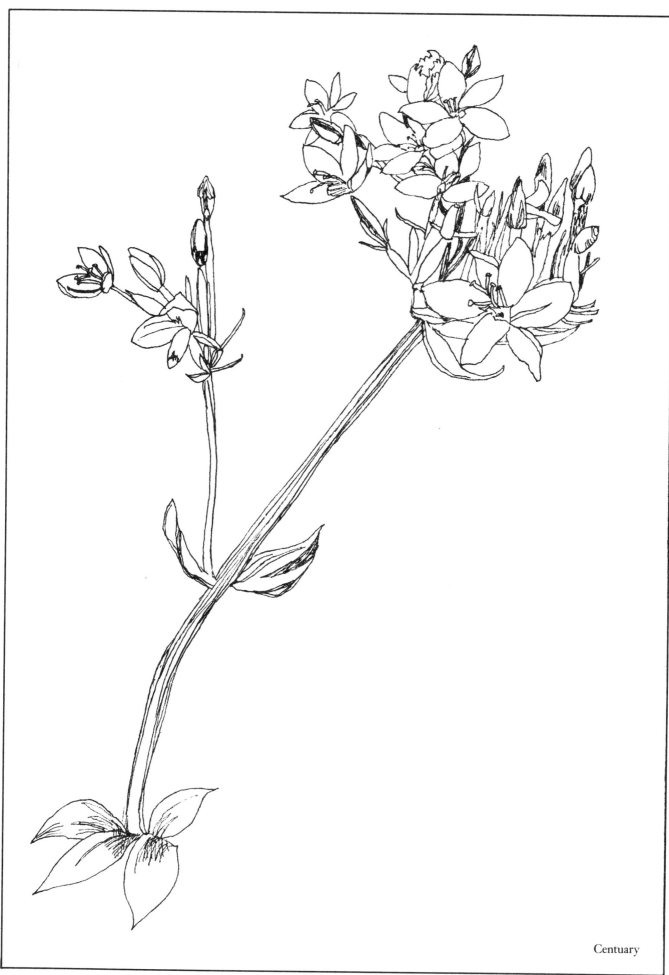

Centuary

CENTAURY

Aliases: Latin name *Centaurium erythaea*. *Centaurium* refers to the centaurs; *erythaea* denotes that it is red. Common names have included Christ's ladder and feverwort.

Companies making the essence: Bach, FES, Healing Herbs, Pegasus.

Essence qualities: The classic Bach profile of Centaury states that it helps individuals who are too easily taken advantage of by others. They are quiet, gentle, submissive, and easily preyed upon by the unscrupulous.

Lore: This herb was attributed to the mythical crippled centaur, Chiron, who was a healer and mentor to Greek heroes like Achilles, Asklepios, and Jason. Chiron was supposedly bitten by a nine-headed poisonous snake called the Hydra and used herbs to cure himself. Witches were said to mix centaury into their incense in order to induce trancelike states. Burning the plants supposedly drove away snakes.

What the plant is like: This pink annual is a member of the gentian family, blooming from June through September. It has clusters of small flowers with five petals and several stamens each, growing on stalks up to 3' (1 m) tall. The flowers prefer the sun, opening in the morning and closing up again at sunset. It grows in dry, sandy soil.

Uses: Herbally, it was used for jaundice, enlargement of the liver, and blood ailments. Externally, it was used for eczema, to treat wounds and as a mosquito repellent.

Reflections: I find that the person who needs Centaury often comes from a dysfunctional family background where boundaries were continually violated. This includes those who have been victims of abuse or molestation.

Affirmations: I STAND FIRM AGAINST PEOPLE WHO TAKE ADVANTAGE.

I RELEASE MY FEAR OF SAYING NO.

I HELP ONLY WHEN IT IS APPROPRIATE.

Astrological correlations: While I have often used it where Neptune is strong, aficionados of the asteroid Chiron feel Centaury is an important essence for difficult Chiron placements, such as to the Sun, Moon, or Ascendant. This association with Chiron, the wounded healer, strengthens my belief that those who need it are often abuse victims.

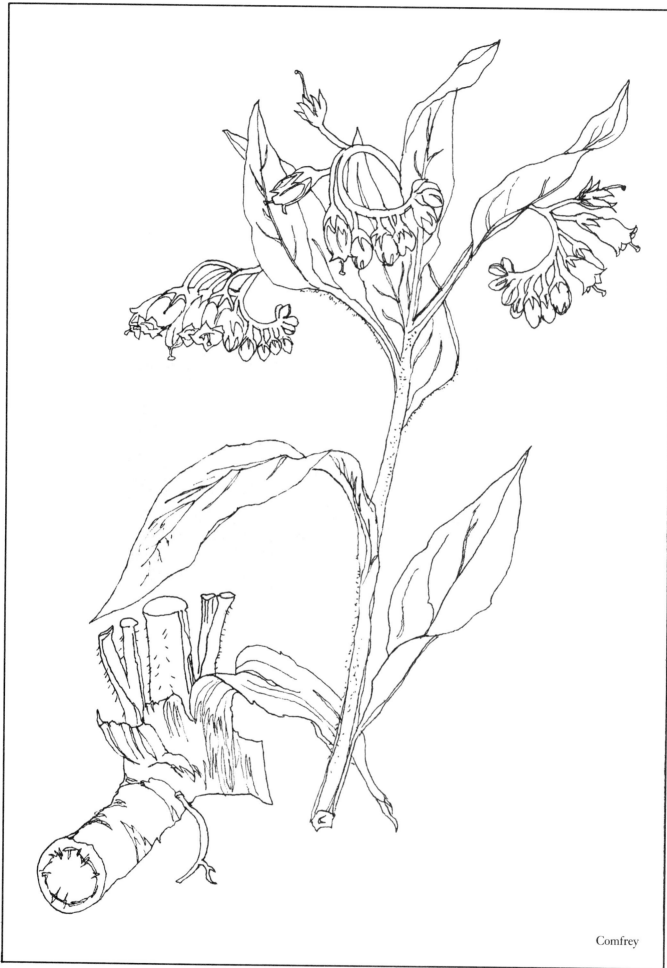

Comfrey

COMFREY

Aliases: Latin name *Symphytum officinale*. *Symphytum*, the ancient Greek name for the plant, derived from *symphysis*—growing together of bones—and *phyton*—a plant. *Officinale* means official or medicinal. Common names include knitbone, boneset, blackwort, gumwort, healing herb, and bruisewort.

Companies making the essence: FES, Harebell, Pegasus, Perelandra.

Essence qualities: The Perelandra description says that it is for repairing higher vibration soul damage resulting from trauma in this or other lifetimes. They recommend you use it in combination with other essences more directly related to the cause of the damage.

Lore: Travelers tucked comfrey in each piece of luggage to guard against theft and in their shoes to ensure a safe journey. It was also used in spells to bring in money.

What the plant is like: The leaves are very large and hairy, and if you touch them, you prickle and itch. It grows on low, wet ground and blossoms most of the summer. The flowers are pale mauve, long, and hollow, growing in hanging clusters of five to twenty. The plant is about 1' (30 cm) tall and 1' (30 cm) wide. The root has a glutinous juice, which is extracted for healing purposes. Unlike most plants, it retains the top growth during the winter; this refertilizes the plant the next season.

Uses: Once nearly universal in gardens, comfrey was grown for centuries as a home remedy. The leaves and roots were crushed as a poultice for bruises, sprains, cuts, and boils. It was used for fractures and taken for a considerable period after an accident to alleviate pain and to heal scars, bones, and tendons. Herbalists used it for hemorrhages and congestion as well.

Reflections: Just as the skeletal system, which is the foundation of the physical form, can be healed by the herb comfrey, so can the essence Comfrey heal the foundations of other levels of being.

Affirmations: I RELEASE ALL DAMAGE DONE BY (NAME EXPERIENCE).

I RELEASE ALL UNWANTED EFFECTS ARISING FROM (EXPERIENCE).

MY SOUL IS IMMORTAL AND INDESTRUCTIBLE; I CANNOT BE HARMED.

Astrological correlations: Comfrey could enhance transits by Pluto, the planet of transformation. It could also be useful in relieving difficult natal aspects by Pluto or Neptune, or any other combination suggesting abuse or trauma.

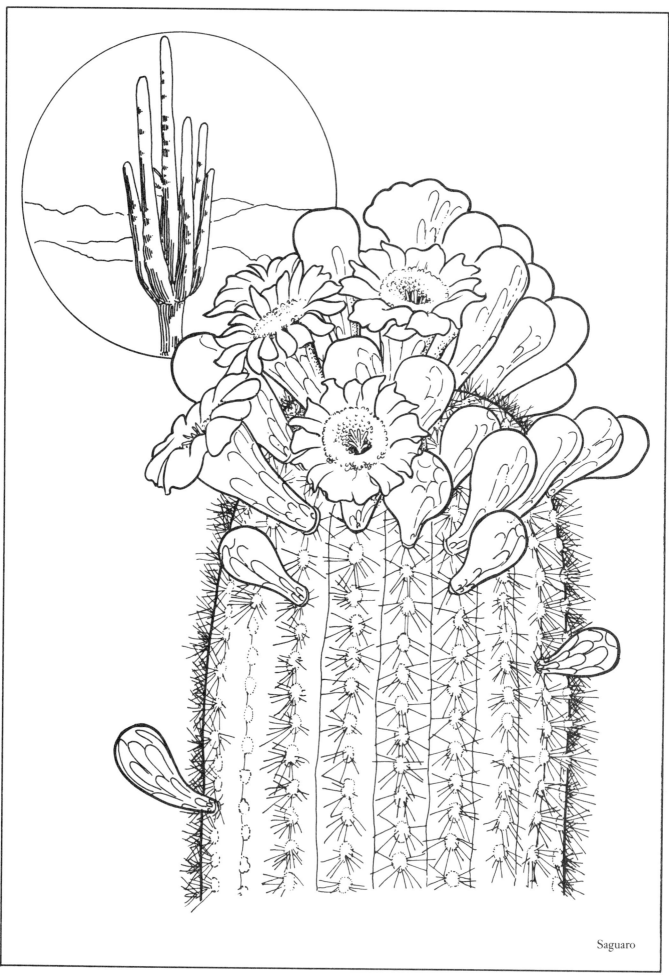

Saguaro

SAGUARO

Aliases: Latin name *Cereus giganteus*. *Cereus* means waxy, *giganteus* means giant.

Companies making the essence: Desert Alchemy, FES, Pegasus.

Essence qualities: FES recommends it for clarity in relationship to authority; for alienation and conflict regarding power figures; appreciation of the wisdom of spiritual elders and ancient spiritual traditions. Balanced relationship to spiritual authority and guidance.

Lore: State flower of Arizona. Undoubtedly, there are Native American legends about this old grandfather of the cactus world, but I haven't found them, nor have the makers.

What the plant is like: Saguaro can become a giant of a cactus, up to 50′ (15 m) high and weighing several tons, although most of the weight is water stored during the short desert rainy season. It can live to be 150 to 200 years old. It is shaped like a huge candelabra, or a man with upraised arms. The large, white flowers bloom for only one day, during the spring rainy season, and then turn to fruits that drop off for seedlings. Though millions of seeds are released, few find good conditions for sprouting and fewer still live to maturity, as they grow only one inch a year.

Uses: It is shelter for many desert creatures, including woodpeckers, which make holes in the trunk. The fruits make welcome food for small creatures. The number of saguaros is diminishing because of poachers who dig them up to sell to florists. Native Americans of the Southwest used the trunks in building homes and ate the fruits.

Reflections: This long-lived plant gives shelter and nurturance to many. It seems like a metaphor for a beneficent elder or authority figure. As it is a desert plant, living solitarily, it may encourage self-reliance.

Affirmations: AUTHORITY ASSUMES ITS RIGHTFUL PLACE IN MY LIFE.

I RELEASE AUTHORITY CONFLICTS STEMMING FROM MY PARENTS.

I STAND IN RIGHT RELATIONSHIP TO TEACHERS AND ELDERS.

Astrological correlations: Saturn aspects to Uranus, Neptune, or Pluto, or aspects by any of these to the Midheaven or the Sun.

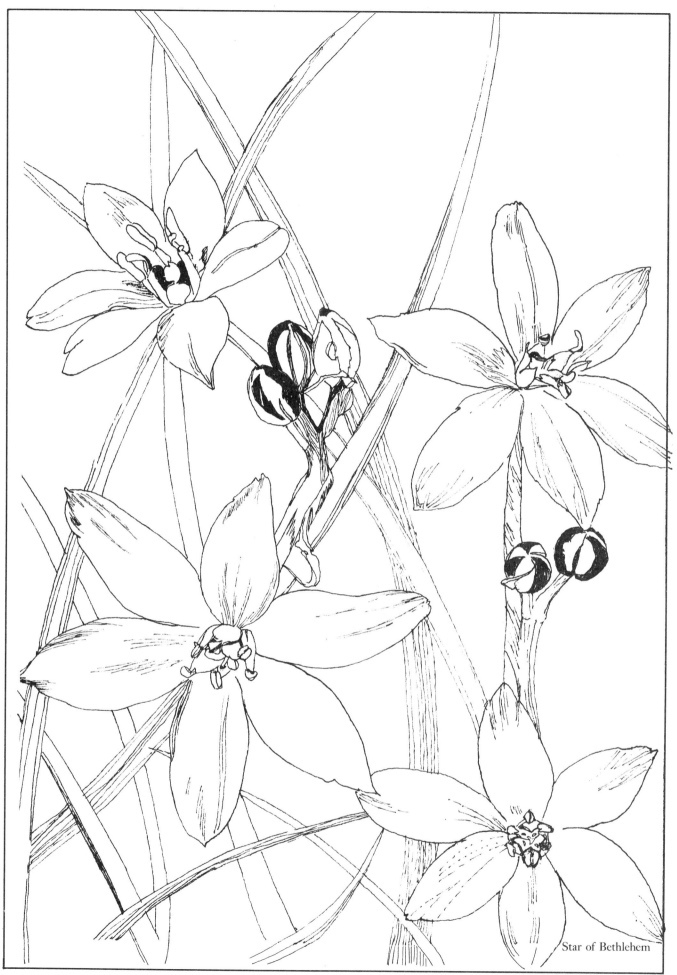

Star of Bethlehem

STAR OF BETHLEHEM

Aliases: Latin name *Ornithogalum umbellatum*. The first part of its Latin name translates as bird's milk; the second means umbrella-shaped. In olden times, it was called dove's dung. It grew in abundance in the Holy Land in the spring and so was given the name Star of Bethlehem.

Companies making the essence: Bach, FES, Desert Alchemy, Healing Herbs, Pegasus.

Essence qualities: For healing shocks and old traumas, no matter how long ago, releasing them from the energy body. Important for victims of abuse, assault, or accidents.

Lore: The bulb was greatly valued in Biblical times, as it could be dug up during famine or siege, roasted and eaten. Sometimes it was dried, ground up, and used as flour. Birthday flower for May 12. In the language of flowers, it signified an afterthought. Elsewhere it was taken as a symbol for unity.

What the plant is like: It grows from a bulb, with long, clear green ribbon leaves, and has a pretty little star-shaped white flower on a 1½″ (3.75 cm) stalk. The bulb is poisonous when eaten raw.

Uses: In Syria and Italy, people still eat the bulbs today, roasted like chestnuts. In homeopathic dilution, it is used against chronic gastric distress and depressed spirits.

Reflections: It was valued during famine and siege, and extreme crisis, and is part of Bach's Rescue Remedy, which is used to help people get through crisis periods.

Affirmations: I RELEASE THE EXPERIENCE OF (NAME TRAUMA).

I AM WHOLE AND FREE OF FEAR ONCE MORE.

MY ENTIRE BEING IS RESTORED TO EQUILIBRIUM.

Astrological correlations: Use during Uranus or Saturn transits or for any configuration in the birth chart showing abuse or life-threatening events, usually involving the outer planets.

Whew! Aren't You Glad That's Over?

No doubt about it—this has been one tough chapter. Topics like these are hard to deal with—hard for the practitioner, and harder still for the person who has lived through them. The excellent self-help books now available can give you an even deeper understanding and appreciation of the vast effects of past woundings. In this chapter, you learned a variety of remedies and tools to help on the long road to recovery. No doubt you will want to come back to them when they are timely. As our next chapter is on relationships, the tools and remedies discussed here may almost be prerequisites for improving the difficult relationship patterns people who have been traumatized often get into.

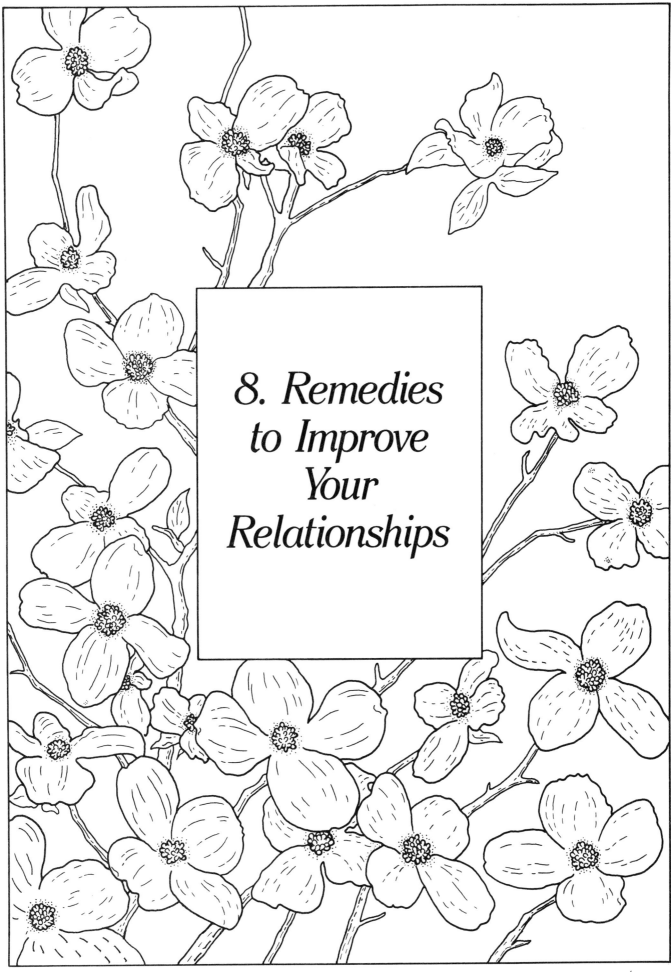

8. Remedies to Improve Your Relationships

You may have wondered why it took us so long to get to the chapter on love. Surely, intimate connection is one of the most important areas of life. When love goes well, it brings us the greatest conceivable joy; when it dies, it hurts more than anything imaginable. Yet, it is only when we are able to cherish and respect ourselves that we attract wholesome alliances. It is only when we make peace with our own emotions that we can cope with the confusing spectrum of feelings that intimacy brings. It is only when we have healed old traumas that we can love without the interference of hangovers from the past. Thus, work in previous chapters prepared the way for this important area. There are many flower remedies to help change the ways you interact. They include some that heal the pain of broken romance and a number for codependency.

We will also discuss some material that is not directly related to flower essences, because in this crucial area a multifaceted approach works best. We'll find additional healing tools for the heart, including crystals, affirmations, and energy work. We'll gain a new understanding of codependency and love addictions as we discover how growing up in a dysfunctional home affects the aura. The remedies and other tools given here for repairing, cleansing, and balancing the heart are crucial to changing painful attachment patterns.

The Modern Relationship Crisis and How It Grew

You have only to look at best-seller lists to realize that partnerships are in trouble. Self-help books like *Women Who Love Too Much*, *Codependent No More*, *Smart Women—Foolish Choices*, *Men Who Hate Women—And the Women Who Love Them*, and *Necessary Losses* sell millions of copies and top the lists for a year at a time. We are going through a period of major turmoil in our most intimate connections, including not only lovers but family and friends.

Where is the difficulty coming from? Many changes in the structure of society contribute to it. It used to be that we were born, lived, and died in the same place, with a large extended family of aunt, uncles, cousins, and grandparents to nourish us. As we become more mobile, in search of success or a better life, we suffer frequent losses and uprooting—either we are moving or those we love are. As the roles of the sexes evolve, and as more and more women work, there are changes in the way we raise children and in the quality of time families spend together. The wars of this century resulted in vast numbers of lost or badly injured fathers and mates. Many who were not outwardly injured were inwardly altered by these experiences.

Divorce is reaching a peak unheard of before World War II. Apart from its impact on the couple, there is new evidence that, even after they grow up, children are deeply touched by divorce. It especially affects self-esteem and their own partnerships. This cannot fail to have an effect, both on programming about involvement and on the capacity to give and receive love.

As we considered while working on self-esteem, the media contribute greatly to dissatisfaction with ourselves and our lovers. Few potential partners can compare to romanticized and surgically enhanced screen idols. Unrealistic expectations of perpetual youth and glamour can lead us to be disappointed with more ordinary mates, with the everyday realities of commitment, and with the hard work of sustaining a relationship. New Age workshops on finding your ideal man or woman and subliminal tapes on how to attract your soul mate tend to perpetuate these fantasies.

All these features play into the current relationship crisis. However, it is useful to understand the positive, evolutionary impulse behind our difficulties. We are increasingly mobile, headed for a time of global consciousness. We are collectively working toward a healthy, whole way for men and women to relate as independent equals, rather than subordinating one sex to another. The two will come together by choice, not by biological and economic necessity. When we compare the legal, medical, educational, and economic status of women and children in the Western world a hundred years ago to what it is today, we can appreciate that we have made great progress. In short, the process is positive over the long haul, no matter how difficult we find this transition period. Meanwhile, you'll be learning ways to heal and strengthen your connections, including some very special flower essences.

The Heart Center and Its Role in Relationships

The key to healing a wounded heart is the heart chakra, which is a real and vital force in closeness. It is located in the same area as the physical heart and is the reason for all those gooey songs about the heart. It is why "the heart aches," why a separation "breaks your heart," and why people say things like "My heart went out to him." The heart center isn't involved just in love affairs. It governs connections with friends, family members, and anyone who touches us in a significant way. When you see an adorable puppy or a darling child and there is a rushing in your chest, that's the heart chakra. When you cry about a tragic death in a movie, your heart has been moved. We call heartless people hard-hearted. This isn't a reference to hardening of the arteries, but to the leaden quality of that person's heart center.

The heart chakra generally develops most when we're in our teens. Up to that time, it has, pre-sumably, taken in nourishment from parental love. The healthy child has had the experience of being loved and even of loving. However, this kind of caring mostly grows out of the fulfillment of the child's needs by the beloved adult. Rather than predominantly taking energy in, the teenager's heart now begins the task of giving more actively to others—of loving rather than being loved. Adolescent crushes, ephemeral as they may be, are the heart's fledgling attempts to open its wings and fly. This stage precedes partnerships based on equal exchange rather than dependency (the root chakra) or ego (the solar plexus). If any of the earlier stages goes wrong, learning to connect in a healthy way becomes difficult. Few people in today's world have had optimal development of their chakras. (Later, we'll see how dysfunctional family patterns affect heart center development.)

Heart Wounds from Broken Romances and Other Losses

When you lose someone you adore, the broken heart of the love songs is all too real. You may feel as if someone stabbed you in the chest. Other separations can leave wounds too—such as the loss of a parent or other cherished family member, especially at an early age, important friendships that are severed, or even beloved pets that die.

Wounds caused by significant disruptions need to be cleansed and healed, or the heart chakra may shut down. So long as old pain, anger, and fear are stuck there, blocking the energy, it's hard for anyone new to come in. You may be afraid of "giving your heart" to others. When the heart is "broken," repair work is necessary.

Part of the repair work—an essential step that cannot be skipped—is letting yourself mourn for as long as you need to. Tears, which contain beneficial enzymes, are cleansing fluid for the heart. If you've never let yourself fully grieve over an important breakup, you may have to go back and finish. It doesn't matter that the affair ended ten years ago. If you haven't been able to love fully since then, blocked-up feelings may still be in the way. Allowing yourself to mourn is one form of healing crisis. You may find it valuable to review the relevant section in chapter 3.

If you sedated yourself with pills, food, or alcohol, as our feel-good society encourages us to do, you froze the grief. It is probably still there in the deep freeze of your emotions, waiting to thaw out, so you can commit totally again. For instance, some people drink hard for many years to avoid experiencing sorrow about a marriage breakup, only to find that, sober, they still have to deal with those emotions. That is one of life's ironies—no matter how hard and how long you run from your feelings, you carry them right along with you!

No doubt this is beginning to sound like hard work, but don't be disHEARTened. It is well worth it, as a heart that is shut down or loaded with grief seldom gets to feel love or joy. Your bonds with others will be more rewarding. You will be able to receive as well as to give. When your heart energy is once more flowing freely, you will experience a richness and fullness in your life, a freedom you may not have known since childhood. When was the last time you felt light-hearted? When were you last able to give yourself wholeheartedly to anything? So, bite the bullet. Have courage. (*Coeur*, the root of courage, is French for heart.) The necessary tools are available.

Seeking Support from Others in Your Heart Healing

One thing you are likely to need in doing this healing is a support network. Undoubtedly, you've partly stopped yourself from grieving in order not to make others uncomfortable. We are given praise for burying our feelings. "She's taking it so well" is an accolade, not a statement of concern. If you're still upset about a divorce or a death three months later, you begin to get feedback like "Isn't it time you let go of that?"

New Age platitudes are even worse. New Age sophomores may ask, in a smug, superior way, "What does it get you to hold on to it?" As you've already suffered a loss, you don't want to risk forfeiting the support of others who are important. You shut up about your sorrow and, ultimately, shut it off.

As you begin mourning, others may again pressure you to stop. You cannot afford to let that get in the way. You need to continue feeling the sadness until it's finished. You can talk to a particular friend or close family member once or maybe twice, but you cannot expect them to listen after that. If you'd gotten their support, you probably wouldn't have closed down to begin with! The longer ago it was, the less validation you are likely to get for your feelings. A traditional psychotherapist can hear you out, validate these feelings, guide the catharsis, and offer a new perspective about what went wrong.

Another beneficial release is to write about your feelings—as long and as many times as seems useful. Some people find it helpful to burn what they've written, with a prayer to let go.

A bereavement group or one for those in the midst of a divorce can be another good place to talk. Even if the parting occurred some time ago, if you're just now dealing with it, it is fresh, and you're entitled. The support of others with similar experiences cuts the isolation and grants permission to deal with all the associated feelings. Members often exchange phone numbers and share their process privately between meetings. Self-help programs can also be an important source of support. (If group participation is difficult, try the remedies given under group work in chapter 4.)

Tools for Mending the Broken Heart

Talk therapy alone cannot completely mend the heart center. Direct work on the energy body and chakras, through flower essences and disciplines like Reiki, MariEl, Polarity Therapy, or Touch for Health, is invaluable. It clears out blockages and gets energy moving again. We've talked about the ways remedy therapy and energy work complement each other, as each works on the aura at somewhat different levels. The combination is especially beneficial to the heart center, since the healing crisis is gentler. You may wish to look for someone who does energy work. When you first begin using the tools given here, some sadness about old losses may come up and be released. You may have some new sensations in that area of the chest. Ultimately you will find that energy flows through it freely and joyfully.

A meditation I have used extensively for heart healing in workshops and with individual clients is one created by Andrew Ramer for our book *Spiritual Dimensions of Healing Addictions*. You can vary it to open and cleanse all the chakras, by using different affirmations. For the heart center, however, visualize a large, closed, many-petalled pink blossom in the area of the physical heart. Use your real hands, not just your imagination, and go around the outside opening the petals one by one. As you do this, say affirmations like: I AM OPEN TO LOVE; I LET LOVE FLOW THROUGH ME AND INTO ME WITHOUT OBSTRUCTION; I AM WORTHY OF LOVE; I LOVE AND RECEIVE LOVE WITHOUT CONDITION; and I AM LOVABLE, LOVING, AND LOVED. Nearer the center, the flower gets warmer and begins to glow with a golden-pink light, which flows from your Higher Self to you. As the center opens, the golden-pink light flows freely down into the heart center, and out into the world. You may need to do this meditation for a while initially and then repeat it from time to time to keep the heart center open through new events.

A gem elixir made from rose quartz in the same way essences are made from plants is mother's milk for the heart center. Rose Quartz elixir is available from Pacific Essences and Pegasus. Dilute it and use it the same way you use flower remedies. Rose quartz crystals themselves are soothing and supportive for the heart center. For healing purposes, you might tape a piece on your heart center or wear a string of rose quartz beads that falls right at the physical heart. Much more expensive jewels, but also beneficial for the heart, are rhodochrosite, ruby, pink kunzite, and pink tourmaline. Can't afford them? They, too, are available as elixirs from Pacific Essences and Pegasus Products.

As gemstones absorb the jangled energy of their users, you need to clear them once in a while. You can clean clear quartz by soaking it overnight or longer in a dish of spring water with sea salt. However, salt leaches color from colored stones. Substitute Rescue Remedy for the sea salt. You might also put the bowl of water with the stones on the windowsill in sunlight. Cleanse them more often if you are working hard on releasing pain.

Anything containing roses is good for the heart center—even if you can afford it, an occasional bouquet. Through the centuries, roses have always symbolized love. Save the petals and dry them for potpourri or use them in a bath. If you have room, grow a bush or two in the yard. Tea rose cologne, the type that smells absolutely authentic, is a loving gift for yourself or anyone else. Aromatherapy oils in rose fragrance are also a subliminal reminder. Put some directly under the nostrils, on the wrist, and behind the ears. Burn a pink, rose-scented candle to change the energy in your room and to heighten meditation.

Flower Remedies for Heart Center Healing

Most essence companies have remedies to cleanse the heart, although here Bach is lacking. However, during what might be called "the dark night of the soul" after a breakup, you'll find that a few days on Sweet Chestnut can be amazingly restorative.

Harebell's Heartsease, profiled later, is a gentle solace and comfort for the broken heart.

Beyond a doubt, the essence Bleeding Heart is unparalleled as a heart healer, but use it with caution. It can initiate a painful catharsis of old hurts and sorrows. The pain isn't caused by the remedy. It has been present all along, but numbed or covered up. Assess carefully whether the person has sufficient ego strength and a good support system to help deal with the feelings. Be sure to explain the healing crisis and what to do for it. It's a good idea to offer a follow-up session or phone call. Perhaps the strong reactions to Bleeding Heart by my clients are not typical, since my practice includes many recovering alcoholics and children of alcoholics. Alcohol abuse has a powerful impact on the heart center.

At any rate, you might want to test for more supportive remedies along with it, such as Heartsease (by Harebell) and Self-Heal. Bleeding Heart is profiled at the end of the chapter.

There are many remedies for heartache. If the need to forgive is part of the problem, the Alaskan Flower Essence Project's Mountain Wormwood is an important remedy, as is the Bach remedy Holly.

Desert Alchemy's Crown of Thorns helps those who believe that they must suffer for love to let go of that belief.

Once the heart is cleansed, you still need to gently reopen it. The Alaskan Flower remedy Alpine Azalea opens the heart to the spirit of love and also increases the capacity for self-love.

They also make Sphagnum Moss, described as releasing judgment from the heart and developing the capacity for unconditional love.

Dogwood, by FES, is quite a special remedy, bringing a capacity for gentleness and grace in relationships. An in-depth profile of Dogwood appears at the end of the chapter.

Mauve Melaleuca, by Living Essences of Australia, brings about a change in both attitude and operating procedures for people who don't feel loved or cared for by those close to them.

FES's Mariposa Lily increases receptivity to human love, healing the feelings of alienation, separation, and being unloved.

Peony, by FES and Pacific Essences, is a beautiful essence I use often for heart center opening. Alexis Rotella says it strengthens the capacity for unconditional love and for not taking others for granted. (See the profile at the end of this chapter.) Peony is excellent to take along with the heart flower exercise on page 124. Dissolve a drop of the essence in a glass of water and drink it slowly.

Fear of intimacy, on both an emotional and a sexual level, is a major barrier to commitment. It takes on many painful disguises, from addiction and attraction to unavailable people, all the way to religious prohibitions against sex.

Sticky Monkeyflower, by FES, is a very important remedy for those who are afraid of intimacy. Their literature also portrays it as good for blocks that are due to unresolved pain about past separations.

Australian Bush Flower Essences offers Wedding Bush, for people who flit from affair to affair, having difficulty making commitments.

FES says that Mallow aids those who create barriers to closeness, bringing about more openness and trust.

For those who are habitually suspicious of people's motives, their Oregon Grape encourages a belief in the goodwill of others.

Where traumatic events resulted in fear of closeness, work with the remedies in chapter 7.

One of my clients was a woman in her late forties. She had married a somewhat older man she loved with all her heart, only to have him incapacitated by a stroke less than a year later. She took care of him devotedly for the next several years. When I met her, she no longer had that day-to-day responsibility, and a very fine and exciting man she had known for some time wanted to be close to her. Although she wanted to be happy about that, she found herself overwhelmed by sadness and a fear of getting involved again. I gave her several mixtures containing remedies like Bleeding Heart, Heartsease, Rose Quartz, and Cayenne, for cleansing emotions. Many sad memories and feelings came up, but she worked through them courageously. Recently, I ran into her with her lover, both of them glowing and quite obviously wrapped up in each other.

Letting Go of Lost Loves

Are you haunted by a lost love? Letting go can be hard, especially when parting involved a betrayal or some other painful rupture. The broken heart, the bitterness, the obsessive thoughts may be all you've got left. And, you may subconsciously believe that so long as you hang on to the pain, you've still got the person in your life. Another unconscious belief may be that, since the person continues to be so important to you, you're still important to him or her, too.

Another, wiser part may also be holding on, however. Sometimes, there is something important that you still haven't learned from the relationship, so you keep replaying it over and over. For instance, you may cling to resentment or sor-

row as a reminder not to let anyone treat you that way again. Inner wisdom may be prompting alertness to the kinds of people who would hurt you. It may be useful to carry on a dialogue, written or mental, with that part of yourself. Ask what it is trying to accomplish by holding on. Have it tell you how to learn or do what is needed in order to let go.

Books on neurolinguistic programming can guide you through this form of dialogue. You might take a look at *Frogs into Princes* and *Reframing* by Richard Bandler and John Grinder, published by Real People's Press. You may also find someone trained in neurolinguistic programming to work with.

As a start, however, it may be valuable to do a written inventory. Include some of the following questions, and if you find yourself resisting them, take some Black-eyed Susan.

- What was the mistaken premise the bond was based on?
- How did you contribute to the conflict or breakup?
- In what ways did you give your power over to your lover?
- In what ways were you or the other excessively dependent?
- How was the relationship a repetition of an old pattern?
- How did your interaction repeat negative family patterns?
- In the long run, would that person have added to or detracted from your continued growth?

We may also return to the 70 times 7 affirmations of Sondra Ray as another writing tool. It is sometimes necessary to do more than one of these affirmations about any given relationship. Some that have proven effective are the following:

I LET GO OF MY ATTACHMENT (OBSESSION, ADDICTION) TO (NAME). (Use Bleeding Heart to help you with this one.)

I FREELY RELEASE (NAME) ONTO HIS/HER OWN PATH. (Use Orchid, for letting go of the past, or Vine, for control issues.)

I AM FULLY HEALED OF THE BREAKUP WITH (NAME). (Bleeding Heart, Sturt Desert Pea, or Heartsease can help here.)

I FORGIVE (NAME) FOR ANYTHING S/HE MAY HAVE EVER DONE TO ME. (Mountain Wormwood helps develop an attitude of forgiveness.)

I ACCEPT FORGIVENESS FOR ANYTHING I MAY HAVE EVER DONE TO (NAME). (Possible essences are Orchid, Mountain Wormwood, and Poison Hemlock.)

ALL THE LESSONS IN MY RELATIONSHIP WITH (NAME) ARE ALREADY LEARNED.

Among the essences, Bleeding Heart is an important tool for releasing painful old attachments.

Australian Bush Flower Essences suggests Boronia for those who are pining for a lost love, with obsessive thoughts about the person, and for a broken heart.

Remedies for letting go of the past mentioned in chapter 7 can also be valuable. For instance, Honeysuckle, by Bach, is for nostalgia. Remember that, historically, honeysuckle was favored for bridal bouquets, so it may have particularly strong implications for relationship nostalgia.

The Alaskan Flower Essence Project offers River Beauty for starting over after a devastating experience.

Pacific Essences provides Poison Hemlock for letting go and not getting stuck.

Essences for Couples in Conflict

Many relationships are essentially positive, even though they may not match the inflated romantic, passionate ideals held up to us by movies, romance novels, and television shows. There are essences to make your bonds even stronger and to help resolve conflicts between loved ones. Ideally, both partners would take the essences; but if even one party undergoes a change in attitude by taking remedies and lets go of hurts and resentments, the quality of the interaction will improve.

Australian Bush Flower Essences suggests Bush Gardenia to couples who are drawing apart because of being busy with their own careers or interests. They find that the essence renews the attraction and interest in the relationship.

Their Wedding Bush is excellent for couples at the beginning of a union or after the initial attraction begins to fade.

FES offers Fig as an aid to developing trust between couples.

Their Basil is said to help resolve emotional and sexual conflict between couples, by facilitating negotiation and penetrating to the essential core of emotional issues.

Dogwood, which we've discussed as bringing increased gentleness and grace in relationships, would be a good remedy for both parties to take, where possible.

One source of conflict is excessive or destructively expressed criticism. Beech, by Bach, encourages a change of attitude in those who are critical and intolerant of others and easily become irritated at their faults.

Calendula, by FES, helps people to be less sharp and cutting in their communications and to listen receptively.

The need to control and dominate, a serious cause of resentment, would be greatly reduced with Bach's Vine. (Why not test for it, even if you're perfectly sure you don't do that!)

You may be wondering whether these essences will save a relationship that is on the verge of ending. Remedies are not a substitute for marital or family counselling, when the differences are great and the interaction between the parties has turned toxic. However, they can support the relationship through increasing communication and awareness of the feelings involved, along with helping to find ways of resolution. When increased awareness brings the understanding that the difficulties cannot be resolved, the combination of counselling and remedies can make the parting less traumatic and more mutually respectful.

If only one takes the remedies and the other is unwilling to do either that or counselling, then the prognosis for resolution is not great. However, the one who takes the remedies will still benefit from the personal growth that the remedies can bring, regardless of the outcome of the relationship. And, as that growth changes the person's attitudes and behavior, the balance in the relationship has to shift along with it.

Remedies for Sexual Wholeness and Role Conflicts

Given all the social changes in this century, both men and women can experience stress in regard to their roles. There are several supportive flower essences.

Men who take FES's Tiger Lily relax excessively aggressive masculine traits, while women who take it often become more assertive. (As we've gone along, you've undoubtedly noticed that many remedies work to resolve either extreme of a polarity.)

Perelandra suggests Chives for the power gained by balancing the male and female aspect of the psyche.

Some essences help to integrate women's struggles for fuller self-development with their equally important need for a close relationship.

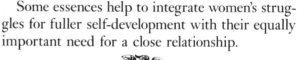

FES characterizes Quince as fostering the positive power of love, especially for women who feel torn between the need for power and strength and the need to be loving and nurturing. (Remember that we discovered quince was probably the fruit Eve gave Adam. As long ago as that, role conflicts existed!)

Japanese Magnolia, by Petite Fleur, allows women to enhance their intellect and talents and to feel independent and secure.

Mala Mujer, by Desert Alchemy, is for women who fear they will express the worst of the feminine archetypes—for example, bitchiness or PMS. (*Mala mujer* is Spanish for "bad woman.")

If there are problems in the sexual area of the partnership—or if the two of you simply want more joy—energy work on the sexual chakra can be very helpful.

Sticky Monkeyflower, a major essence for those with fear of intimacy, is especially valuable for sexual fears.

Balsam Poplar, by the Alaskan Flower Essence Project, fosters release of pain and emotional tension associated with sexual issues.

Basil, by FES, alleviates conflicts between spirituality and sexuality.

Alexis Rotella says that Peony, in addition to all of its salutary effects on the heart, can bring ecstasy to the act of love.

Desert Alchemy offers a Sexual Harmony formula, which both partners may take.

Wisteria, by Australian Bush Flower Essences, is for those who are uncomfortable with sex and intimacy, especially the macho male.

Living Essences recommends Macrozamia for women's problems around sexuality.

Some words of caution are in order. Please note that these remedies are not "love potions." They do not create an attraction where none exists. Be aware, also, that what appear to be sexual problems in a relationship are often only a smoke screen for deeper conflicts between the two parties.

One of my clients had finally gotten married to a man she'd been involved with for many years. When she returned from the honeymoon, she confided that she was now experiencing some sexual difficulties with her husband. When I suggested Hibiscus essence, she mentioned that on their honeymoon, in the Caribbean, she had been fascinated with the voluptuousness of the hibiscus flowers she saw everywhere. I wish I could say she took Hibiscus and lived happily ever after. Instead, although she felt an increase in sexual energy, she became clear that her husband treated her in certain ways that turned her off. These behaviors were connected to long-standing conflicts that being legally committed had only exacerbated. With this new clarity, they addressed these issues in marital counselling.

The Dysfunctional Family and Its Effects on the Heart Center

A major cause of chronic relationship difficulties is growing up in a dysfunctional family. Impairment generally starts in childhood, when family members don't give the child a feeling of love-worthiness. Alternately, these interactions may make the child feel that caring has too high a cost, so that he or she is frightened to accept it. Many of us have been affected by the bogus forms of affection our parents gave us that left us feeling unloved—e.g., substituting food, candy, or possessions for quality time together. Above all, growing up in a family where addictions are present powerfully affects a child's adult relationships.

In *Further Dimensions of Healing Addictions*, my coauthor, Andrew Ramer, and I discuss how ad-
dictions massively damage the aura, which needs to be healed as part of recovery. Sugar and alcohol are closely related chemically and have a similar effect on the heart center, so they have important consequences for relationships. On a physical level, these two substances bring a rush of blood to the heart, so it feels as though the heart chakra has opened, moved, and filled up, even though it has not. Heavy drinking or sugar abuse often begins after a divorce or a broken romance, as people try to fill the emptiness. It doesn't work for long. The abuse of either alcohol or sugar or both progressively numbs this center, causing it to shut down.

The frozen heart center cannot accept love,

OUACHITA TECHNICAL COLLEGE

even when it is freely given, so love is not felt and cannot be returned. More and more isolated as a result, alcoholics or sugar addicts try desperately to get love. They learn to manipulate others and to make people pity them. They feel a rush of energy into their hearts when someone else's heart goes out to them.

When alcoholics or sugar addicts stop using their substance and enter a twelve-step program, the center may still not thaw out. It usually must be opened and restored consciously. In support groups, there is a powerful, healing fellowship, but not everyone can connect with it. When there is major damage to the heart chakra, many people remain isolated or form twisted alliances, even in recovery. Some individuals simply shift addictions, changing from alcohol to sugar or to sex and love addictions. The remedies and other tools discussed in this chapter can help to heal the heart and change the addictive pattern.

How Mates and Children Are Affected

Addiction creates *energy imbalance* because there is no *energy exchange*. This affects the heart centers of the addict, his or her mate, and their children as well. The distortion is progressive. Even after that person leaves or gets sober, the imbalance tends to become established as an energy exchange pattern in later attachments. Thus, repairing and nourishing the heart chakra and other important parts of the energy body are crucial to the recovery of the addicted and those who care for them.

In the addicted family, the sober parent transmits to the children sorrow, rage, and a desperation to cure the alcoholic. This becomes the role model for the child. The addicted parent transmits intoxication along with love energy, so the child feels an intensity that it identifies as love and comes to expect in intimacy. As an adult, he or she is drawn to alcoholics or addicts because they provide the "heart highs" that ordinary relationships seldom reach.

Given the way they grow up, many adult children of alcoholics (ACAs) may wind up living what they learned, which is to turn to alcohol or sugar to stimulate the heart center and fill the emptiness they feel. In those who are already susceptible, loss of a loved one may trigger alcoholic drinking or sugar binges. In women, serious weight gain often begins with marriage and the birth of children, as they are called upon to give abundantly of heart energy they themselves never received.

Even in recovery, the addicted ACA may switch to love addictions, using other people as the drug of choice. Damage done to the solar plexus in a dysfunctional home and/or during the addiction also needs to be repaired, or the person will continue in self-hatred. Look back at the remedies given in chapter 5, particularly Sunflower and Alpine Azalea—they are also important in recovery.

Even when the ACA or adult child of a dysfunctional family doesn't turn to addiction, the heart chakra can present difficulties. With their combination of low self-regard and overdeveloped heart centers, many feel good about themselves only when they are able to rescue or serve others. This is why ACAs tend to get involved with one alcoholic after another throughout life. Many ACAs or adults from seriously dysfunctional families seek careers in service fields such as psychotherapy, health care, astrology, and various forms of healing. Red Chestnut and Centaury, both by Bach, can help keep service and self-nurturance in balance.

Codependency as a Consequence of Heart Center Distortion

The term "codependency" derives from the field of chemical dependency, and it is generally applied to the families and "significant others" of people with addictions. It also applies to those whose lives are significantly affected by the illness or dysfunction of those they care for. Codependency is an addiction to the addict or some other dysfunctional person. The obsession with curing or changing them grows and is perpetuated as a pattern of bonding. Almost all untreated ACAs form codependent relationships of one kind or another, or stay away from codependency by staying away from commitments.

In his important and readable book, *A Primer for Adult Children of Alcoholics*, psychiatrist Timmen Cermak delineates the following common characteristics. Codependents change who they are and what they are feeling to please others. They feel responsible for meeting other people's needs, even at the expense of their own. They have low self-esteem and are driven by compulsions. They also have the same use of denial and distorted relation-ship to willpower that is typical of active alcoholics and other drug addicts.[1] They find it easier to focus on their loved one's problems as a way to avoid looking at their own.

Energy work through such tools as Reiki and flower remedies can contribute significantly to recovery from codependency, as can bodywork. By clearing and rebalancing the overdeveloped heart chakra and the underdeveloped solar plexus, a healthy new pattern of energy exchange in relationships may be more easily established.

Remedies for Codependency

Certain flower essences are especially good for codependents—and for practitioners working with them. For balance between relationships and one's own needs, you would need to combine them with essences for self-esteem.

We've spoken of Bach's Rescue Remedy. However, I've also designed "the Rescuer's Remedy"—one that offsets the compulsion to rescue and save people. The contents of this combination vary slightly, but it generally includes Bach's Chicory, for those who are always trying to set others straight, and their Red Chestnut, for those who suffer excessive anxiety for others. Pine, Bach's remedy for guilt, helps them to feel good about taking care of their own needs. Centaury, by Bach, is for those who are too easily taken advantage of or have a history of victimization. (For the person who has actually been a victim, the work in chapter 7 may need to come first.) If you're a rescuer or are working with some, try the Rescuer's Remedy.

Rhubarb, profiled later, is described by Harebell as for people who have problems with their own or others' boundaries, especially for those who intrude on others.

Desert Alchemy provides a combination formula called Making and Honoring Boundaries, which has proven very effective.

They also offer Bright Star, for those who can't say no.

Red Clover, by FES, helps to keep a person centered while others are going through emotional upheavals. (We noted earlier that the Druids valued red clover for psychic protection.)

FES's Sagebrush is for being true to your essential self and not overidentifying with others.

Living Essences of Australia offers Straw Flower Everlasting for people who feel so depleted they have nothing left to give.

Very often, the problem in establishing boundaries began on the psychic level. If you are at all psychic—and, certainly, all of us have that potential—test for Yarrow in order to shield yourself from bombardment by other people's feelings and needs.

Desert Alchemy recommends Wild Grape for those who experience enmeshment rather than healthy boundaries, defining themselves by their relationship to those around them.

Harebell's Cymbidium helps people to stand up for themselves and releases them from their fear of others' disapproval.

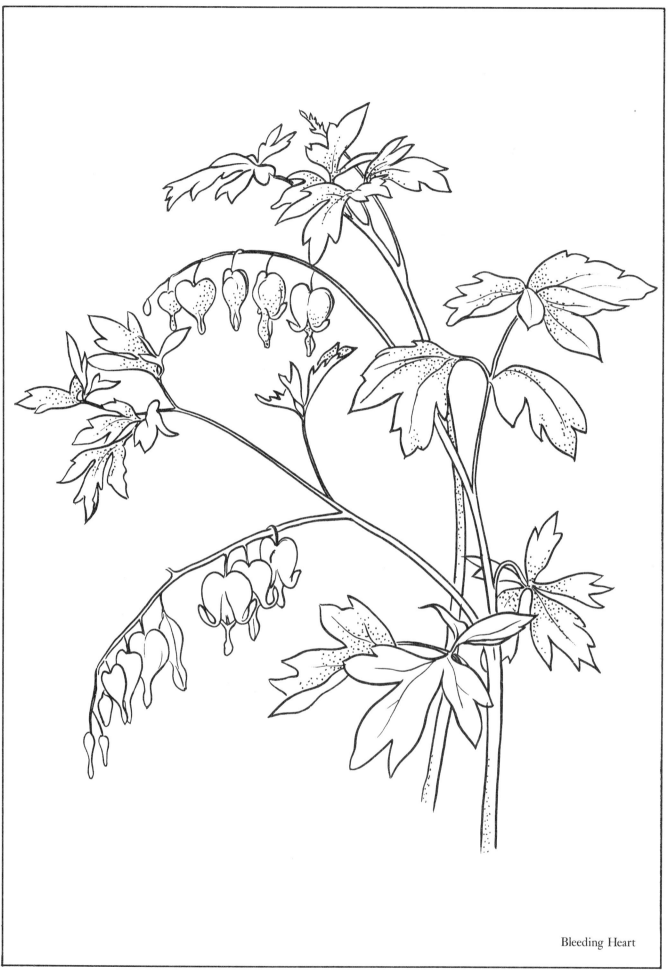

Bleeding Heart

BLEEDING HEART

Aliases: Latin name *Dicentra formosa*. *Formosa* means beautifully formed. *Dicentra* means it has two spurs. It was also called locket flower, for the shape of the blossoms. (Many lockets are heart-shaped, and hold pictures of those we love.)

Companies making the essence: FES, Pegasus.

Essence qualities: I find this essence a powerful heart center cleanser and healer, but use with caution, as it can produce strong catharsis. The FES description says it is excellent for releasing painful emotional attachments and heartache over a broken relationship; and that it brings peace, harmony, and balance to the heart. Also for those who are too clinging, possessive, or overidentified with those they love.

Lore: Bleeding Heart was originally found in Japan and China. It was used as a love oracle—crush the blossom, and if the juice is red, the person in question loves you; but if it is white, forget it! It was considered unlucky when grown indoors, but if you put a coin in the pot, it changed the luck.

What the plant is like: Colors go from red to bright pink to white. Six to ten delicate heart-shaped blooms hang from a slender, arching stem that grows up to 2½″ (6.25 cm). At first, the heart is intact, then as the blossoms grow larger, the tips begin to open and a white teardrop protrudes. They can be grown successfully only in moist, cool, shady habitats, as they shrivel up with too much sun or heat. These perennials can be grown from seed or root division.

Uses: Infusions of the roots have been used by some herbalists as a tonic and diuretic, but it is not widely recognized as an herb.

Reflections: That the blossoms hang (depend) from the stem suggests that unnecessary dependency will cause heartache. Pink is the color of love, and red of passion, so the necessary healing colors are present in the flower. The drop that drips from each blossom is a reminder that tears are healing for the heart.

Affirmations: I RELEASE MY ADDICTION/OBSESSION WITH (NAME).

I RELEASE THE PAIN OF MY BROKEN RELATIONSHIP WITH (NAME).

MY HEART IS HEALED, WHOLE, AND OPEN TO LOVE.

Astrological correlations: Use when Venus aspects Pluto, Neptune, or Saturn in the birth chart, or when you find Pluto, Saturn, or Neptune in the seventh house. It also helps when Pluto, Neptune, or Saturn transit Venus or a seventh house planet.

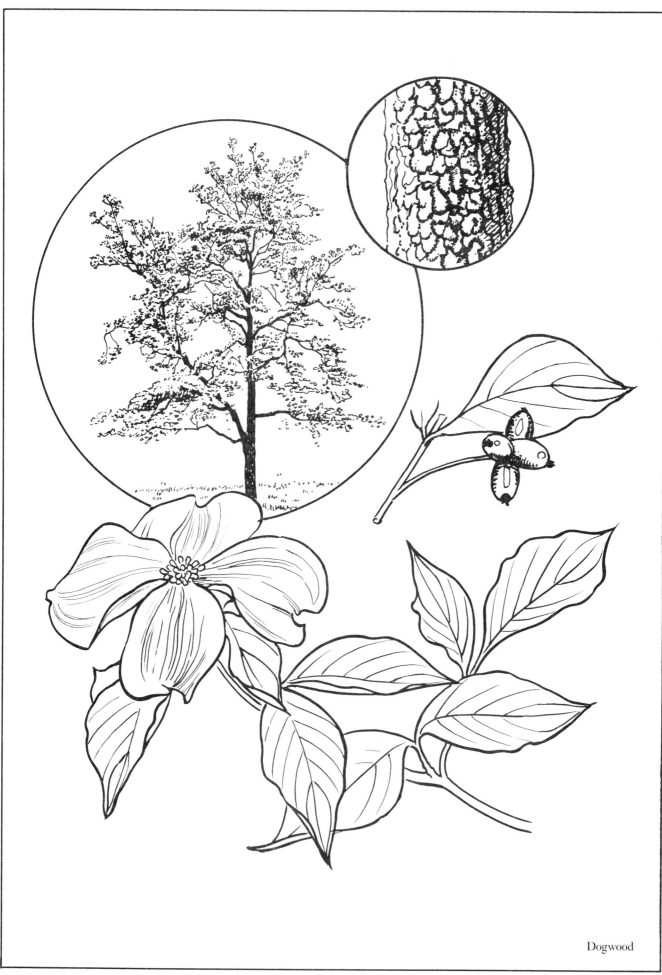

Dogwood

DOGWOOD

Aliases: Latin name *Cornus nuttalii*. *Cornus* (horn) and *nuttalii* (for botanist Thomas Nuttall). Common names include boxwood, cornel, and dog tree.

Companies making the essence: Desert Alchemy, FES, Pegasus.

Essence qualities: The FES catalog says Dogwood is for gentleness and grace in relationships and the etheric body. It also assists clarity of emotions while attuning to spiritual sources. Eases hardening of emotions and attitudes associated with past trauma or abuse.

Lore: In the language of flowers, it means "love undiminished by adversity." It symbolizes beauty, faithfulness, and stability. Magically, it was burned before important meetings to ensure a positive outcome. The leaves were carried in amulets for protection. Widely admired in the American South, it was named state flower of Missouri and Virginia.

What the plant is like: The dogwood tree has a showy composite bloom, with a head of tiny green flowers in the middle and four large, spectacular, white to pink petals surrounding them. When the outer petals fall, the tiny green flowers in the center develop into a cluster of small red, fleshy fruits that stay on the tree into autumn. The bark is like the skin of an alligator. The tree ranges from 16′ to 40′ (5 to 12 m) in height.

Uses: Formerly used medicinally as a mild astringent and tonic, it sometimes served as a substitute for quinine when that was not available. The wood is next to hickory in hardness and was used for the shuttles of the loom. Native Americans boiled the roots and washed down muskrat traps with it; the animals were attracted by the dogwood scent.

Reflections: Dogwood trees are among the hardest of woods, yet Dogwood essence is an antidote against hardening of the heart and the etheric body. The symbolic meaning of love undiminished by adversity seems reflected in the essence descriptions.

Affirmations: I TREAT MYSELF AND MY LOVED ONES GENTLY.

ALL HARDNESS OF MY HEART IS DISSOLVED.

I RELEASE ALL TENSION CONNECTED WITH LOVING.

Astrological correlations: The remedy strengthens natal Venus in any of its signs, but especially when Venus is in aspect to Saturn, or when Saturn is situated in the first or seventh house.

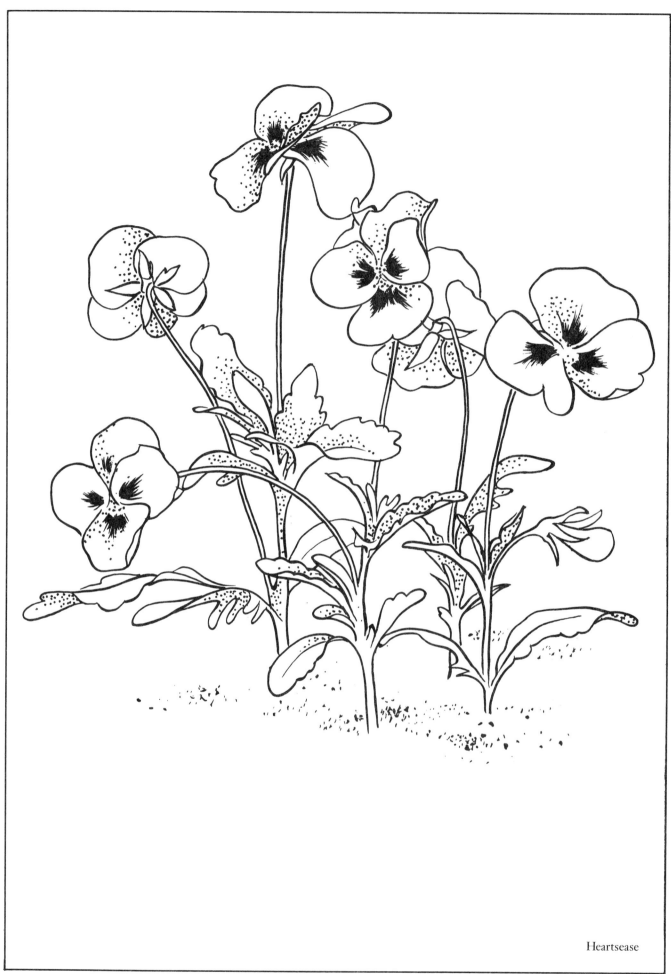

Heartsease

HEARTSEASE

Aliases: Latin name *Viola tricolor*, meaning a three-colored violet. Commonly known as herb trinity, as the three colors in one flower reminded people of the Holy Trinity. Also called Johnny jumpups, wild pansy, tickle-my-fancy, or love-in-idleness.

Company making the essence: Harebell.

Essence qualities: The Harebell literature says it eases broken or damaged hearts, hurt, or loneliness. Brings comforting thoughts. I use it frequently for gentle heart center healing.

Lore: The flower was once used to make a love potion. Shakespeare blamed it for Titania's falling in love with an ass in *A Midsummer Night's Dream*. People believed that by carrying the flower about with you, you could ensure the love of your sweetheart. The name of its tame relative, pansy, came from the French word *pensée*, which means "thought," so in the language of flowers it meant, "You are in my thoughts."

What the plant is like: It is a member of the violet family. A perennial miniature wild relative of the pansy less than 2" (5 cm) across and about 1' (30 cm) high, it has multicolored petals in purple, yellow, and white.

Uses: Its medicinal properties were known in the days of Hippocrates. It was used to cure venereal disease. It was also considered to have beneficial effects on heart conditions and high blood pressure. Herbalists used it for bronchial, skin, and rheumatic conditions.

Reflections: There is a sweetness and joy about these little flowers. The lore and the healing uses all confirm the connection between this flower and the heart center.

Affirmations: MY HEART RELEASES ALL SORROW AND IS WHOLE.

I AM GENTLE AND LOVING WITH MYSELF AND OTHERS.

I ATTRACT KINDNESS AND LOVING PEOPLE TO MYSELF.

Astrological correlations: For those with difficult natal aspects to Venus, such as Venus/Saturn or Venus/Neptune or difficult seventh house placements. Also comforting for recent difficult transits to Venus or seventh house planets.

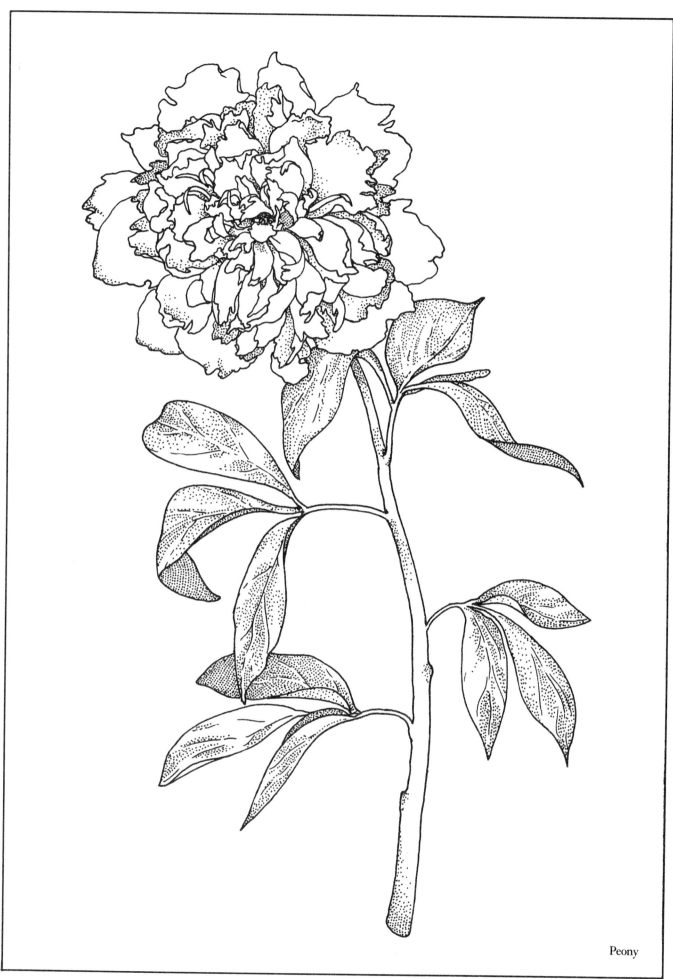

Peony

PEONY

Aliases: Latin name *Paeonia officinalis.* Taken from the name of Paeon, a healing deity of ancient Greece whom Homer called physician of the gods, and who first taught man about the medicinal properties of this plant. *Officinalis* marks this as a medicinal plant. Old common name was piney.

Companies making the essence: FES, Pacific Essences, and Pegasus.

Essence qualities: Alexis Rotella says that it is excellent for heart center opening, unconditional love, not taking people for granted, creative blocks, and bringing about God-intoxication.

Lore: A legend holds that Paeon was given the plant on Mount Olympus by the mother of Apollo, the Sun god. Alexis Rotella points out that this flower was cultivated in China centuries ago and can live to be as old as a hundred years. The Chinese considered it the king of flowers; it symbolized abundance to them. Flower for June in the Japanese flower calendar. In Europe, mischievous nymphs were said to hide in the petals. In the Middle Ages, the seeds were strung as a necklace and worn to keep away evil spirits. When gathered in the moonlight, it was supposed to be a cure for lunacy, and was also used to exorcise imps and incubi. In the language of flowers, it means shame or bashfulness. Birthday flower for June 21. State flower for Indiana.

What the plant is like: A low, softly bushy plant 3′ to 4′ (1 m) high with large leaves and big, striking, white, pink, or red flowers. They bloom from May to August, depending on the climate. Once planted, the peony does not like to be disturbed, and refuses to flower for several years after transplantation.

Uses: The root has been used medicinally to reduce muscle spasms or tightness, to induce vomiting, and as a strong laxative. The seeds were also thought to bring on menstruation and to relieve gynecological difficulties. Peony was thought to have narcotic properties and was widely used against epilepsy. It was said to relieve nightmares and sad dreams.

Reflections: This is one of my favorite heart center remedies, a rather intoxicating heart-opening.

Affirmations: I LOVE MYSELF AND OTHERS WITHOUT CONDITION.

I RELEASE THE FEAR OF LOVING AND BEING LOVED.

I ACCEPT THE LOVE OF THE DIVINE AND THE DIVINITY OF LOVE INTO MY LIFE.

Astrological correlations: Peony is a remedy that helps heal all difficult Venus aspects. It seems especially good for Venus aspects to Neptune or to Neptune placements in the seventh house.

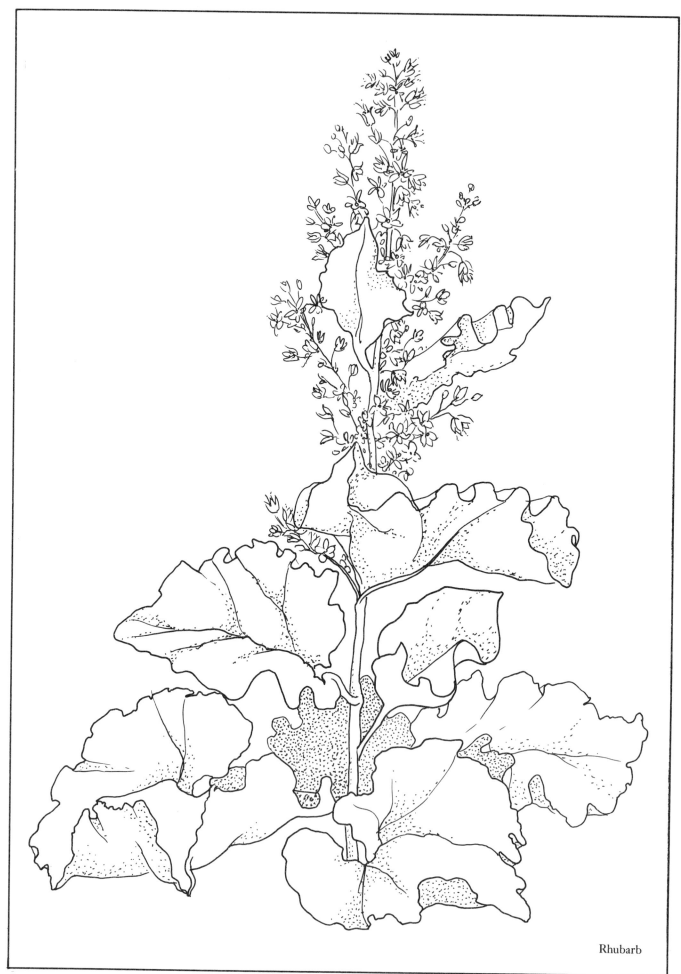

Rhubarb

RHUBARB

Aliases: Latin name *Rheum*, from the Greek common name for rhubarb, *rhēon*. The common name was pie plant, for its most common culinary use.

Companies making the essence: Alaskan Flower Essence Project, FES, Harebell, Pegasus.

Essence qualities: Harebell recommends it for problems with your own or others' boundaries such as insecurity, vulnerability, being way off center, exhibitionism or talking too much.

Lore: Women made it into pies to keep their husbands from straying. Birthday flower for May 25. Symbolized advice.

What the plant is like: Rhubarb belongs to the smartweed family and originally came from Mongolia. It is a vegetable, not a fruit. The stalks are up to 2′ (60 cm) tall, thick and reddish-green, each topped by a single large, umbrella-like leaf. Only the stalks are edible; the leaves are poisonous. The plant lasts five to eight years, and is best planted from roots.

Uses: As food, it was cooked in pies and stewed. The roots have the most medicinal properties. Both roots and stalks were used as a mild laxative, which was especially helpful for infants because of its gentleness. It was also given to them for colic. Rhubarb was widely used as a tonic, particularly for the liver, thyroid, and gall bladder, for bad breath, and as an astringent. It was also said to dissolve blood clots and relieve earache. Cosmetically, women used it to strengthen their nails and, steeping the stalks with honey and wine, to lighten their hair.

Reflections: The tartness of the plant, which must be liberally sweetened with sugar, seems likewise significant of relationship issues, as does the fact that only the stalks are edible and the leaves are poisonous. That's about boundaries, all right!

Affirmations: I KNOW WHERE I BEGIN AND OTHERS LEAVE OFF.

I RELEASE THE NEED TO MERGE WITH OTHERS (OR, NAME).

I RESPECT MY LIMITS AND THOSE OF OTHER PEOPLE.

Astrological correlations: As Neptune astrologically relates to the issue of boundaries, anyone with a strong Neptune might want to test for this essence.

A Word of Encouragement for the Weary!

We've taken a hard look at relationships in today's world and the difficulties connected with them. In order to heal ourselves of losses that we feel we have suffered, we may need to relive sad, difficult feelings and experiences. Remember to work at your own pace, leaving it when you've had enough for a while, then coming back when ready to unload even more. Gentleness with yourself in this process is a good preparation for accepting gentleness from others. The payoff for perseverance is a new freedom in loving others and being open to receive love in return. Released from the burden of old sorrows, our hearts will be lighter and more capable of experiencing joy. Ideally, our partners and other loved ones will undertake their own heart healing, perhaps in part through some of the essences mentioned here.

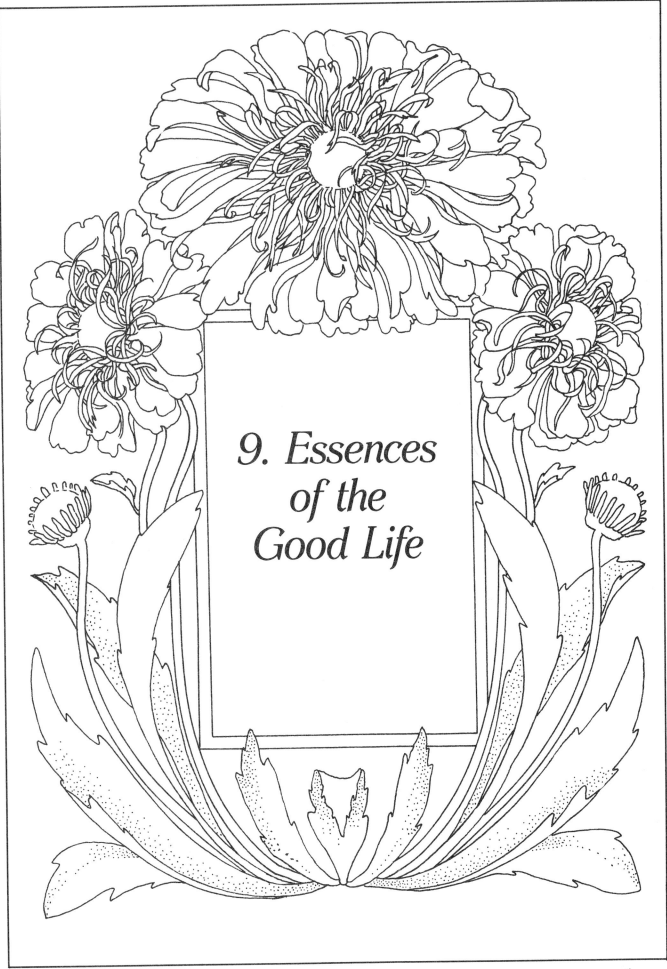

9. Essences of the Good Life

We've worked on so many difficult things that by now you may wonder whether the remedies have anything to do with happiness. Indeed, they do, and you're going to learn about some beautiful ones now. However, in order to get to joy, you may first need to start clearing out accumulations of painful emotions and sorrow over past events and people. It may be necessary to begin reopening the heart center and coming to love yourself. Please notice nothing is being said about completing these processes, only beginning them. The sequence is something to come back to again and again, as you are progressively more able and willing to release these old burdens.

With this chapter, we get to the good part. We're going to discuss essences for career success, creative self-expression, spiritual development, playfulness, and an increased capacity for happiness and abundance. Don't put off taking these remedies until you've finished your karmic housecleaning. It's helpful and uplifting to take some at the same time you're releasing painful memories or scouring the solar plexus of self-hate.

For instance, by taking Zinnia, for playfulness and laughter, you might be surprised to find yourself laughing at parts of the process.

Or, after taking African Violet, for love and nurturing from the Higher Self, you might feel a strong sense of support from this eternal part of your being.

Finding Your Life Direction

One of the most important ingredients in happiness is finding and honoring your life direction. When you're doing the things you were born to do, life is deeply rewarding. Resisting these things is like walking through molasses. The trick, of course, is finding what those purposes are—and they may be different at different stages of life.

When we were children, we knew. Those silly things we told our parents we were going to be when we grew up may not have been so far off the mark. After all, the word "silly" comes from the Middle English *sely*, which means good, blessed, or innocent. It may be useful to remember those earlier choices and find a way to do some of them now. Unless they are hopelessly grandiose, you may be able to do them on a lesser scale. We can't all be movie stars, but you can participate in local theatre productions. We can't all write best sellers, but surely you could write a piece for your local paper, for starters.

Among the Bach selections, Wild Oat is a constitutional remedy for those who are unfulfilled and dissatisfied because they haven't found their goal in life. Melanie Reinhart, an excellent flower remedy teacher in London, says that unfulfilled people want to achieve something special, but have only the vaguest notion of what that might be. They have difficulty committing to a vocation, because they don't want to do things the traditional way. They suffer from creative unrest, trying many things and finding many opportunities, but getting bored with everything after a while. Wild Oat types are usually unconventional, multi-talented people who haven't found their niche. The popular expression "sowing wild oats" usually refers to a young person who isn't ready to settle down. The Wild Oat individual may carry this restlessness far beyond youth. Taking the remedy, perhaps more than one bottle, can make a difference.

The Australian Bush Flower Essences include two that are helpful in these instances. Silver Princess, which is more for the person under the age of 28, brings an awareness of one's life direction for those who are despondent and aimless. At other times, it helps people at a crossroad see what the next step is. Or, after reaching an important goal, Silver Princess may ease the commonly felt letdown by giving a glimpse of what's next and restoring motivation. It also makes it possible to enjoy the journey while striving for the goal.

Their Red Lily is for people over the age of 28 who feel scattered, disconnected, split, and lacking focus. Indecisive daydreamers who take this essence become grounded, focused, and live in the present. (The astrologically sophisticated, of course, will recognize the age of 27 to 30 as the Saturn return, when we are finally true adults.)

Desert Alchemy says their formula, Connecting with Purpose, facilitates defining and integrating your purpose into daily life.

Fulfilling Your Divine Mission, another of their combinations, is said to help you do what you came here to do, so you can be fulfilled.

FES features Mullein for listening to inner guidance and fulfilling one's true potential, especially for people who know their purpose, but whose talent or goal has not gained recognition. Also, Mullein supports people in holding on to an unusual or difficult vision despite a lack of social validation. (Mullein, profiled in chapter 5, is a complex and useful essence.)

Walnut, by Bach, is excellent for people in transition. It has proven essential after major career or geographic moves, to help people feel settled and grounded again. A woman who suddenly relocated from the East Coast to California found that she needed it continuously for six months. Any time the dosage bottle was empty and she forgot to refill it, she began to feel confused, unfocused, and paralyzed.

Desert Alchemy's Transitions Formula is proving useful for similar needs.

FES's Blackberry is recommended for those who are overwhelmed by the magnitude of their goals and who doubt their ability to manifest them.

Their Tansy, profiled in this chapter, helps people to take decisive action toward their goals, particularly when the right course of action is known but lethargy or procrastination arise.

A Life with New Direction

So far, we've seen only snippets of case histories. The difficulty is that most clients who come to me for ongoing work have multiple, difficult issues. Many are from dysfunctional and often abusive backgrounds and may be recovering from an addiction or two. Thus, there is seldom any neat resolution of single issues. Besides our work, they are often referred for traditional therapy, twelve-step programs, health care, and energy work. With so many new factors operating at once, it can be difficult to tell what part the essences play in a person's recovery.

Recently, however, I have seen a very clear-cut and satisfying example of a substantial change in direction in just three months through remedies alone. A man, let's call him David, came for a chart reading the week of his thirtieth birthday. (Yes, astrologers, it was his Saturn return.) He was depressed because he no longer wanted to work in sales, wasting time on something that didn't provide growth. He had no career plans, and his self-esteem was low, but he felt he had to make a move.

From his chart, it was clear David had fine potential as a healer, probably in bodywork or nutrition. Having been involved in yoga and other spiritual studies for many years, he was pleased to hear this. He was most inclined toward nontraditional training. Since he doubted his abilities, I gave him Buttercup, so that he would value his own gifts and get over feeling he wasn't good enough, and Alpine Azalea, for loving himself.

When David returned six weeks later, he wanted to apply to chiropractic college, but was holding back because his last educational experience had ended badly. He was given Bach's Gentian, to release an old setback, their Larch, for those people who believe they will fail—and therefore fail to make the effort—and Transitions Formula to move through this transition period more easily. I repeated Buttercup and Alpine Azalea. I also suggested he get concrete information about requirements by checking catalogs from different schools.

At the next appointment a month later, David had overcome the old educational barriers and was actually enrolled in some needed math and science courses. Now he was wavering between chiropractic college and an acupuncture course. I suggested he visit a local chiropractor who had an acupuncturist on staff, to talk to them both. I gave him a new mixture containing Bach's Scleranthus to help with the decision. As usual, I included Buttercup and Alpine Azalea.

On the last visit, he had decided on an acupuncture course and was moving forward confidently. He also requested something to improve meditation. Alpine Azalea no longer tested positive, but Buttercup did. I also gave him Australian Bush

Flower Essences' Cognis Formula to help with the science courses, the Alaskan Flower Essence Project's Polar Ice for completing cycles, and Lotus for meditation.

The contrast between the depressed, self-doubting person David had been just three months earlier and the radiant, confident person he was on this last visit was wonderful to see. No new elements had been added to his life, only the essences and, of course, the encouragement and practical direction from our once-a-month sessions. Beyond a doubt, his innate gifts, his ability to work with suggestions, and his motivation for change were also key factors. However, he had had the same gifts before beginning this work, but was paralyzed by self-doubt and despair.

Remedies That Help Develop Attitudes and Habits for Success

Many people have a good idea what their special gifts and purposes are, yet have trouble getting started on that path. They may be overwhelmed at the difficulty of the task or may not know exactly how to begin. Then, there's always inertia, the resistance to movement that drags down all animate and inanimate objects.

FES's Blackberry is a fine remedy for helping you overcome inertia and translate your thoughts into action.

Their Madia stimulates follow-through and focus.

Their Trumpet Vine helps you project yourself actively and dynamically, with the kind of vitality that enlists others on your side.

The Anchor-Manifestation Formula by Desert Alchemy is useful for making dreams and visions a reality.

They also offer Cliff Rose for those who are unfocused and unable to follow through on some creative idea or project.

Cytisis, by Harebell, helps people keep moving despite distractions, difficulties, and lack of help or encouragement.

Some life tastes are so difficult that the individual may become overwhelmed. The tools for self-esteem can assist you to gain the confidence to move onward.

Additionally, in the Bach kit, Elm helps those who are capable, yet sometimes feel inadequate to the task or weighted by responsibilities.

I often use two FES remedies for people who are overwhelmed by difficult tasks. As the catalog describes, Penstemon works against self-doubt, and Scotch Broom replaces despair and pessimism with faith and confidence. *The Flower Essence Repertory* recommends the use of Scotch Broom for despair over external blockages—say, the world situation—rather than one's own limitations. The outcome of taking this remedy is that the person begins to see obstacles as opportunities for growth and service to the world.[1]

Negative attitudes work against success, and there are many remedies against them. Perelandra's

Okra is for the gloom-and-doom type who sees everything in the worst possible light. Several others are specifically restorative when you're trying hard to realize a vision, and you run into blockages.

As mentioned before, Larch, by Bach, strengthens and motivates people who believe they are going to fail, so they don't even try.

Borage, by FES, is also strengthening for the discouraged, bringing confidence and cheerful courage.

Bach's Gentian is often described as being helpful for people with a negative outlook, who become discouraged easily and quit. However, I have found that this type of discouragement often takes hold after a bad setback or series of tough breaks—sometimes long ago. It then carries over into subsequent situations. For example, it has often been helpful for performers who haven't even been able to bring themselves to audition in years. On examination, they often admit that they stopped after some devastating failure or humiliation, finding themselves "blocked" thereafter. Gentian, especially when combined with energy work on the solar plexus and other chakras, has helped them begin anew. If you've run into a block with your particular vision—say, to start your own business—test Gentian.

Bach's Gorse is for even deeper despair, when you've made strenuous efforts, tried many things, and nothing has worked.

The final stage in this spectrum is resignation and apathy: The individual no longer even cares. This type becomes passive and chronically bored, believing that circumstances can't be changed. For this state of mind, Bach's Wild Rose can result in a new lease on life.

The depressing effects of an overwhelming long-term struggle or long-term despair can be relieved by Australian Bush Flower Essences' Sunshine Wattle. In Ian White's beautifully written and illustrated book on their essences, *Australian Bush Flower Essences*, he recommends it for those who have had a difficult time in the past and who are stuck there, carrying those negative experiences into the present. They see life as a grim struggle, bleak and hard, with no sense of future success. Sunshine Wattle returns optimism and joyful expectation, with acceptance of the beauty of the present.[2]

I had been giving a variety of remedies for months to a woman who was deeply dissatisfied with her life. She wanted to leave the city, but was unable to do anything about it. She was extremely negative, ending each session with a litany of complaints about how bad everything was and how much worse it was getting. She seemed to enjoy this song and dance, but I was becoming a bit discouraged. I added Sunshine Wattle as the only new remedy in the mixture she was taking. There was a distinct shift in her attitude. She began to mobilize herself to take action and even allowed a little laughter in the sessions.

Sometimes our visions run into barriers because there is a lack of understanding or validation from important others or from society. Sometimes there is even active opposition. Cymbidium, by Harebell, gives the strength to confront and defy undermining influences and to overcome the fear of disapproval.

FES suggests Trumpet Vine for self-assertiveness.

Their Mountain Pride is described as lending strength and assertiveness in the face of adverse forces, resulting in spiritual warriorship and positive masculinity to face challenges.

Essences for alienation, like Shooting Star or Mariposa Lily, may also be comforting to those whose vision is long ahead of its time. Remedies such as these allow us to take greater joy and fulfillment from our work.

Liquid Assets—Remedies for Prosperity

There are also essences that bring about the attitude changes necessary to allow more prosperity. True prosperity is not to be confused with conspicuous consumption. A major lesson for both nations and individuals in the Nineties is about the illusory and ephemeral nature of status and affluence based on unwise borrowing and overspending. We're beginning to recognize the prevalence of debt compulsions, addictive spending, and credit card abuse.

How can we let go of the illusion of wealth and find a path toward real financial stability? There are many good metaphysical tools for prosperity. Energy work such as Reiki on the root chakra and possibly the solar plexus may be helpful. Sondra Ray's technique of writing a statement 70 times a day for seven days can be helpful at getting at the roots of poverty consciousness. Try statements such as these:

MY SELF-ESTEEM IS SEPARATE FROM MY FINANCIAL STATUS.

I RELEASE ALL BARRIERS TO A GOOD INCOME.

I RELEASE ALL PARENTAL CONDITIONING ABOUT MONEY.

I RELEASE MY ATTACHMENT TO STRUGGLE AND DRAMA.

I RELEASE MY FEAR OF FINANCIAL INSECURITY.

I GIVE UP COMPULSIVE SPENDING.

I STOP BUYING THINGS TO MAKE MYSELF FEEL BETTER.

I USE CREDIT SANELY.

There are also flower remedies for working through barriers to sound financial health. Even though the Bach kit was developed during the Great Depression, none of those remedies seems specifically aimed at prosperity. Oak, however, relieves the feeling of a long, hard struggle, especially where there have been serious financial concerns over a period of time.

FES's Star Thistle is suggested for stinginess and an inability to share, which often comes from a fear of lack. It opens the personality to abundance rather than the need for outer security.

An excellent remedy is Polyanthus, which Pacific Essences recommends for dissolving blocks that get in the way of abundance and for transforming attitudes of scarcity into ones of worthiness and willingness to receive.

Pacific Essences also offers both an Abundance Essence combination and an Abundance essential oil. The founder, Sabina Pettitt, has designed a 21-Day Abundance Program using both of these combinations, as well as affirmations and actions for each of the 21 days. Preliminary results are excellent.

Desert Alchemy features a Celebration of Abundance combination.

Both fascinating and useful in sorting out attitudes that limit prosperity is Money Plant by Pegasus. The plant, which is often used in dried bouquets, has seeds that look like silver dollars. In her fine book *The Essence of Flowers*, Alexis Rotella shows how this essence gives insight about the barriers to prosperity and helps change attitudes that stand in the way. I've given it to many clients and find them getting smarter about money. Several of them suddenly decided to put their credit cards away or tackle long-standing tax problems.

Essences for penetrating illusion may help the individual see the truth about debt financing. They include Sand Dollar by Pacific Essences, which is not a plant but a sea creature, and Bladderwort by the Alaskan Flower Essence Project.

Bach's Cherry Plum helps break destructive habits of whatever kind, especially when you know what you're doing is bad for you, but can't resist.

Remedies to Alleviate Stress, Fatigue, and Overwork

Chronic tension and stress make it hard to enjoy life. Dandelion is helpful for those who strive too hard and overstructure their lives. FES sells it in both massage oil and liquid form.

Their Garlic is also good for nervous tension and insecurity.

Their Dill counteracts the overstimulation that comes along with the fast urban pace of life and so often leaves people feeling overwhelmed.

When work is chaotic and fast-paced, with the need to juggle many demands at once, their Indian Pink increases effectiveness.

The Universe Handles the Details is a delightful combination by Desert Alchemy. It facilitates giving up the need to control the minutiae and surrendering personal will to the direction of Universal will. The name alone is a healing!

Nothing can rob people of the zest for life like unrelenting fatigue. It is important to note that exhaustion may have many medical causes. These include chronic infection or systemic viruses, cardiac or pulmonary insufficiency, or adrenal exhaustion, which can come from constant stress or caffeine abuse. Deep fatigue can also be a symptom of either chronic or acute depression, which we discussed in chapter 6. It is important for the individual to have a checkup to ascertain if fatigue is due to a medical condition or clinical depression and to follow up on any required treatment. Flower essences are not a substitute for necessary health care, exercise, and proper diet, all of which have salutary effects on exhaustion.

Where health problems are not at fault, deep fatigue may be a consequence of unrelenting stress and overwork. The Bach kit contains several remedies for this pattern.

Hornbeam is for that draggy morning feeling, the kind that goes away after several cups of coffee.

When people take Hornbeam for a while, they seem able to cut back on caffeine without conscious effort. This remedy is specifically for those who do too much mental work, living in their heads, and whose fatigue is mainly mental.

Next in degree is Olive, for people who are both mentally and physically exhausted and have been for a long time.

Finally, comes Oak, for those who keep on striving despite long hardship. At some point, especially at midlife, this type of person may be overcome by fatigue, for which Oak is a great solace. Sometimes more than one of these remedies is required. (Oak will be profiled at the end of the chapter.)

When we discussed the healing crisis, we spoke of the badly exhausted woman who took a mixture for fatigue and had to go to bed for several days. This reaction was seen as a healthy one, because she had been pushing herself unwisely into a collapse. The chronically fatigued, overworked individual may take a mixture, rest and feel better, then go right back to the old pattern. Another crisis may come up, another mixture for fatigue, another crash. This may happen a few times, especially if the person does not continue taking the remedy after starting to feel better. Ultimately, the person gets smarter, changes the pattern of overwork, and perhaps makes corrections in diet and exercise as well.

Besides the indispensable Bach remedies for fatigue, there are some useful contributions by other companies. FES's Aloe Vera is important for restoring burned-out life force energy.

You may also wish to test their Tansy, profiled later, which helps overcome sluggishness and lethargy.

The Alaskan Flower Essence Project offers several remedies they class as elemental, not made from plants but from the unique environment of Alaska. One of these, Portage Glacier, is for cleansing and revitalizing.

Desert Alchemy has a combination formula called Unwind—Integrating Being and Doing, which they say helps with relaxation, especially for workaholics who "do" in order to escape being present.

They also suggest Whitethorn for those who are driven, exhausted, overextended, or burned out. After taking it, people learn to be more gentle with themselves, to prioritize, and to use their energy in a new way.

Enhancing Your Creativity

Working in New York City, I see many creative people in my astrology and therapy practices. It is a work of joy to support them in expressing and expanding their gifts. Three of my favorite remedies are often in the picture here.

A variety of makers agree that Iris, profiled later, is excellent for creativity. FES suggests it is most helpful in overcoming blocks and a feeling of limitation. A stained-glass iris hangs in the window of my consultation room, as an ever-present evocation of the iris plant angels.

The second of the triumvirate, Indian Paintbrush, is described by FES as awaking the vitality of the creative impulse. They also say it develops vigorous forces of will in those who have difficulty supporting the intensity of creative work.

The third, Buttercup, is not for creativity per se, but it is particularly helpful to those whose creativity is blocked by self-doubt or undervaluing their abilities. (You may have detected my partiality to this sweetheart of a remedy!)

I gave this combination to a painter who came for an astrology reading. He was intensely frustrated because he couldn't seem to paint. Old material and techniques were no longer rewarding to him, and he was stagnating. Six weeks later, he wrote to say he'd had a breakthrough. He claimed the remedies had worked wonders, and he wanted a refill. Enclosed was a photograph of the first of his new creations—a glorious, vividly colored, stylized painting of an iris!

I have recently acquired Desert Alchemy's Creativity Formula, which puts us in touch with inspiration and also helps us stop judging our efforts and thus blocking them. It will be interesting to see how this one differs from the others.

Calendula, which is FES's remedy for knowing the power of one's words, has often been effective with writers.

Writing, in part, comes from the throat chakra, with its connection to speaking out, and working on the throat chakra with essences and energy can remove blockages. Trumpet Vine may be useful when writing about a cause or strong viewpoint.

Harebell's Cymbidium, for overcoming the fear of disapproval, helps when the creative person is bucking the popular trend and adopting a style that is unpopular or not yet validated.

Several of the companies address the problem of creative block. All too often, blockages arise from the emotional content of the work, which the writer or artist is having difficulty confronting. Remedies for emotional integration like Fuchsia or Scarlet Monkeyflower may be needed.

When the block follows a bad review or other setback, Gentian helps put the disappointment or sense of failure behind you.

FES also recommends California Poppy for creative blockage, but does not explain the connection. With this remedy's primary purpose being for those who need glamour or "highs," I suspect it is more for addicted or recovering artists than for other types.

We've been talking about people everyone would agree are artists, but what about you? Do you recognize your own gifts, and are you using them to enhance the quality of your life? Many of you are saying, "But I can't draw or put a sentence together on paper." Perhaps not, but don't limit your definition of creativity to the fine arts. Improvising a recipe is creative. So is rearranging your living room in a pleasing new manner. Making costumes for a Halloween party or choosing new accessories for an old outfit require creativity. Wrapping presents and arranging flowers are forms of self-expression. *Webster's Dictionary* defines creative as "bringing something into existence out of nothing; originating; making."

If you still think you lack talent, take Buttercup for a while, then follow up with Iris. You may very well surprise yourself and add great pleasure to life in the process.

Happiness, Vitality, and Zest

A loving gift to give yourself would be FES's Zinnia for lightness, joy, and release of tension. The catalog says it results in a childlike, playful attitude toward life and improves the relationship to the inner child. I often add Zinnia in the midst of work on heavier concerns, and it is like adding sunshine.

The Desert Alchemy combination formula called A Way to the Elf helps when we take ourselves and our purposes too seriously. It expands consciousness to a state of pure simplicity, lightheartedness, playfulness, and hope.

Desert Alchemy also offers Strawberry Cactus, for those who take life too seriously and don't have fun. It allows them to let joy and fun into their lives.

Harebell suggests White Narcissus for becoming acquainted with the child within. It helps us let go of the rigid superego and move from our heads to our feelings.

Australian Bush Flower Essences advises Little Flannel Flower both for children who are too serious and for adults who need to regain their playfulness and join in play with their children.

They also recommend Sunshine Wattle, described earlier for those who've had a difficult time in the past and assume the present will be just as hard. Taking the remedy returns optimism and joyful expectation, with the acceptance of the beauty of the present.

FES features California Wild Rose for vitality, rejuvenation, and overcoming apathy. They say it restores enthusiasm and positive involvement in life.

I have often used their Nasturtium to restore earthiness to the person who lives in the head and has little vitality.

If someone needs essences for fatigue, however, it may be necessary to take them before going on to the others.

Remedies for Spiritual Growth

In a certain sense, all remedies promote spiritual growth. As we leave behind outdated emotional habits and relationship patterns, as we come to love ourselves, and as we release painful past experiences, we grow spiritually. We reconcile with our fellows and come closer and closer to the beings we were meant to be. You can't hate others or yourself and love Spirit wholeheartedly at the same time. If everyone on the planet took Holly, Willow, and Pine, the collective release of negativity and hate would be so profound that the kingdom of heaven would be at hand! Still, meditation, dream work, and other spiritual practices can be strengthened by several flower essences.

For those who are new to the spiritual path or who may be experiencing a dry period upon it, there are some very fine offerings.

Just as the lotus blossom has been an important spiritual symbol for centuries among many different religious groups, the remedy Lotus, profiled later, is one of the finest for spiritual growth.

As a remedy of infinite tenderness, I often include African Violet, which Petite Fleur says touches a chord within the spirit to release nurturing and love from the soul and Higher Self.

Bush Iris, by Australian Bush Flower Essences, stimulates spiritual awakening and opens people up to spirituality and to the door of their higher perceptions. They say it is excellent for those who have just started meditation or conscious spiritual growth, because it cleanses the root chakra and opens the crown.

When entering the spiritual path and at various points in the process, it is natural to grapple with the question of one's connection to the Divine. Where the relationship with the earthly father has been troubled, there is almost always a reverberation in the relationship with the Eternal One. Since we inevitably confuse the two, rarely is the spiritual path without potholes, detours, and false turns for those who have grown up in alcoholic or severely dysfunctional homes. (See Chapter 7.)

Often, the problem is not so much with the Divine, but with the messengers, to whom such people transfer that need for an all-knowing, all-loving parent. They look for godlike qualities in those who seem to be in touch with the Divine. When the messengers themselves are ACAs, the potential for distortion is compounded.

FES's Saguaro, profiled in chapter 7, is helpful in healing troubled bonds with the earthly father.

Taking it can have the unexpected benefit of bringing the relationship with the Eternal Father into better perspective as well. Saguaro provides balance in relationship to spiritual authority and guidance, with renewed appreciation of the wisdom of spiritual elders and ancient spiritual traditions. When dealing with gurus or teachers, it is an important support.

FES portrays St.-John's-Wort as lending trust in divine protection and guidance. Magically, it was used as an herb of protection, especially during thunderstorms, and tossed on fires and burned.

Remember that flowers with the name of lady were dedicated to Mary, although many of these same plants had pre-Christian associations with the Goddess. Lady's Mantle, by Harebell, is for those who seek the protection and inspiration of the Goddess.

There is often a tendency for beginners to rush from one teacher or fascinating study to another—from reincarnation to shamanism to astrology to the tarot—winding up with the spiritual and mental equivalent of indigestion. FES's Shasta Daisy is an unparalleled essence for this stage, as it helps you synthesize knowledge gained from all these sources into a whole embracing diverse ideas or perspectives. (The flower shasta daisy is shown on the title page of this chapter.)

While immersed in the lofty realm of spiritual studies, it is crucial to stay grounded. Bach's Clematis, described as being for "space cadets," has often been indicated for spiritual disciples.

FES suggests Corn for attaining a balanced relationship between heaven and earth, the spiritual and the material.

Their Manzanita is also for groundedness and being at home in the body. They especially advocate it for those who have a deep-seated or unconscious revulsion to the physical body or earthly realm.

Essences to Support Spiritual Practices

Flower essences and dream work go hand in hand. While taking any remedy, you may have dreams that clarify the nature of the problem and help work through experiences and emotions related to it. It is especially useful to take one of the daily doses before going to bed. However, for those who wish to use dream work as a part of their path of growth, there are specific remedies.

Magically, mugwort was considered an important protective herb. It was burned as incense. It was used in making dream pillows, which people would sleep with to gain visions of the future and important spiritual insights. Similarly, FES suggests Mugwort for greater awareness in crossing the spiritual threshold, especially during sleep.

Any mixture is stronger when combined with affirmations and creative visualizations. It is best to take a dose just before you do them, with a clear intention formed in your mind.

FES's Madia helps bring visions into manifestation, and they particularly recommend combining it with Blackberry and Iris—a trio they nicknamed "The Manifestation Formula."

There are remedies for those who wish to develop psychic abilities in a whole and balanced way—or for those who are already psychic, but feel bombarded by the input they're receiving. FES's Star Tulip stimulates psychic awakening and receptivity to the inner voice.

In my experience, this essence is best combined with Yarrow. That Yarrow is made by at least six companies testifies to its importance. FES recommends it for psychic shielding and strengthening the inner light, so that you are not vulnerable to harmful influences. Yarrow, an herb with a very long history, is profiled later.

Fringed Violet, by Australian Bush Flower Essences, protects people who work with psychic skills.

As psychic abilities develop, there is a human tendency for ego to get attached to these experiences. We forget that it is within the capabilities of most human beings to have intuitive perceptions, even though most people block them in all but moments of crisis. It is precisely when ego becomes involved that abilities like channeling are least reliable. Sunflower may be a helpful antidote to this tendency, as it develops a healthy, balanced ego and self-esteem.

FES recommends California Poppy for those who seek outside themselves for spiritual "highs."

Some essences for the spiritual development defy categorization. The Alaskan Flower Essence Project has taken advantage of a unique environment to make some unusual remedies.

Northern Lights, made under the Aurora Borealis, helps us reach beyond ourselves into the unity of the universe. It cleanses and repatterns our energies, especially around the heart.

Polar Ice is for times of transition and the completion of cycles, so that you can better understand the rhythms and subtleties of time.

Solstice Sun helps one create and maintain a channel within for the free flow of light and energy, especially for integrating peak experiences.

Among their plant essences, Green Bells of Ireland allows us to feel at home on the earth and to live in a more balanced relationship to it.

Their Labrador Tea makes it possible to center energy in the moment and in the body.

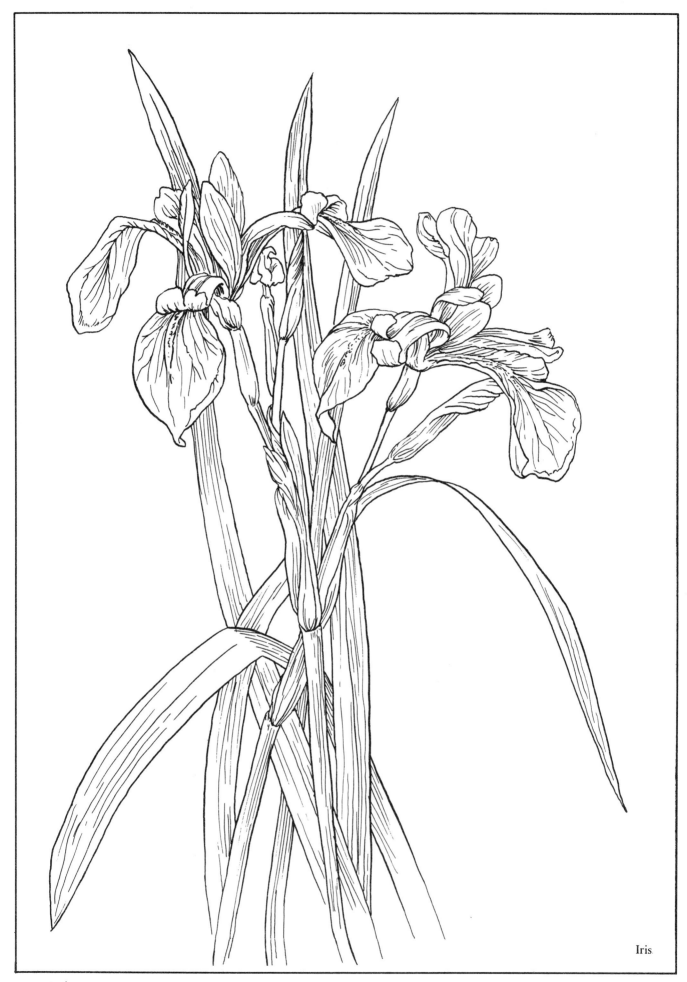

Iris.

IRIS

Aliases: Latin name *Iris*; named for the goddess of the rainbow, Iris. Common names were orris or blue flag.

Companies making the essence: Alaskan Flower Essence Project, FES, Petite Fleur.

Essence qualities: The various makers agree it is for creativity.

Lore: Associated with the rainbow goddess, Iris, it symbolized hope and the eternal spirit. The plant was often used as a funeral herb. The flower was said to bring peace to the departed and to ensure a good life in the next incarnation. Iris was also sacred to the Egyptians as a symbol of the Pharaoh. Perhaps because of this association, the royalty of France stylized it as the fleur-de-lis and took it as their emblem. It's the Japanese flower of the month for May. In the West Indies, the whole roots, which resemble the human form, were used in voodoo spells, and the powdered root was an ingredient in love potions.

What the plant is like: There are many gorgeous cultivated versions of the iris, although remedies are generally made from the simpler wild version. All operate on a plan of three—three petals, three sepals, three stamens, and three styles. (Thus, various religions used it to symbolize three in one.) The plant stands 2′ (60 cm) high, with blooms 3″ (7.5 cm) in diameter.

Uses: When the roots are dried for about two years, they smell like violets. They were widely used in perfumed powders, foot powder, soaps, and cosmetics, and still are to this day. In the days when people were more fearful of dampness, the powdered root was used as a dry shampoo. Orris root is still a fixative in potpourri, a remnant of the time it was used magically in incense as an herb of protection.

Reflections: This lovely flower inspires our love of beauty and stimulates the brow and crown chakra. Those who try it will have a new appreciation of their own brand of creativity.

Affirmations: I EMBRACE MY CREATIVITY IN ALL ITS FORMS.

I RELEASE ALL NEGATIVE INPUT ABOUT MY SKILLS.

I DRAW UPON DIVINE INSPIRATION ALWAYS.

Astrological correlations: Brings out the positive potential of Neptune; also strengthens fifth house planets and Venus.

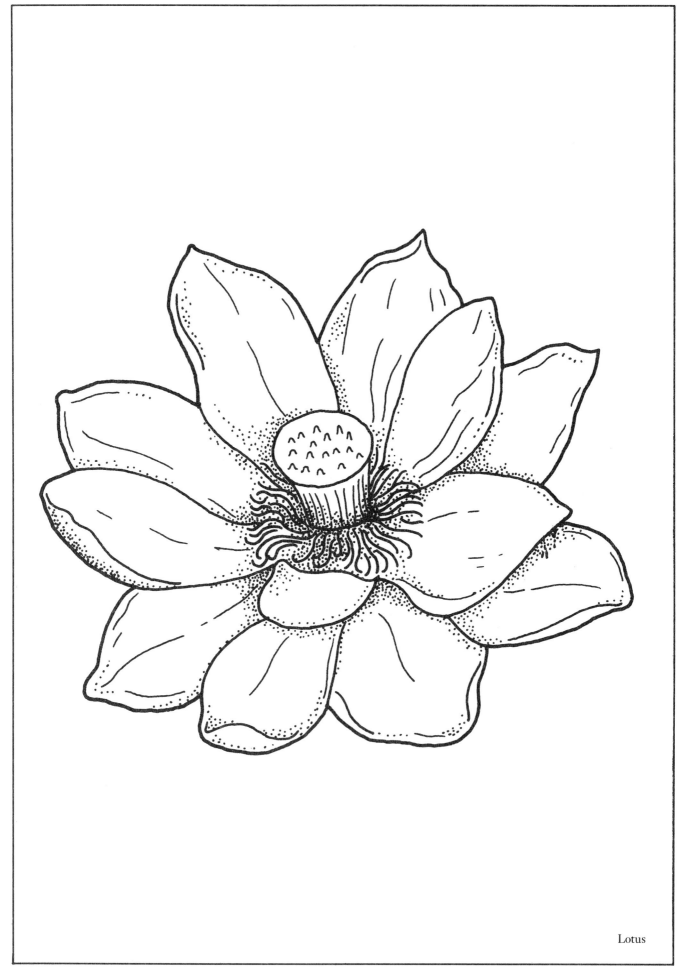

Lotus

LOTUS

Aliases: Latin name *Nelumbo nucifera*. *Nelumbo* was the old Ceylonese name; *nucifera* means nut-bearing.

Companies making the essence: FES, Pegasus.

Essence qualities: A major essence for all phases of spiritual development and spiritual studies.

Lore: The lotus has been considered a sacred symbol in a variety of religions for over 5000 years. For example, in ancient Egypt it was a reminder of resurrection, because the flower closed its petals at night and sank beneath the water. It then reemerged and opened its petals again with the morning sun. Buddha is often pictured seated in the center of a lotus. Magically, the seeds were an antidote to love spells. In the language of flowers, it meant eloquence. Birthday flower for November 9.

What the plant is like: A water plant, with huge blue-green leaves shaped like an umbrella. The awesome single, white blossoms, sometimes tinged with pink, are as big as 10″ (25 cm) across. In the center of the blossom is a flat-topped receptacle that contains many nutlike seed capsules.

Uses: The pod was used as an incense burner, and the oil was also used in meditation. The seeds are edible and are propagated by Oriental people for food. The seeds can sprout after being dormant for centuries.

Reflections: The fact that so many cultures revere this as a holy plant corroborates the spiritual qualities attributed to the Lotus essence. Test it for all who have an interest in spiritual studies; it corrects or prevents the many imbalances that can develop.

Affirmations: I DELIGHT IN MY CONTACT WITH THE DIVINE.

I EMBRACE THE DIVINE IN MYSELF AND OTHERS.

THE SPIRITUAL AND MATERIAL ARE ALWAYS IN BALANCE.

Astrological correlations: Balances Neptune and brings out its positive potentials.

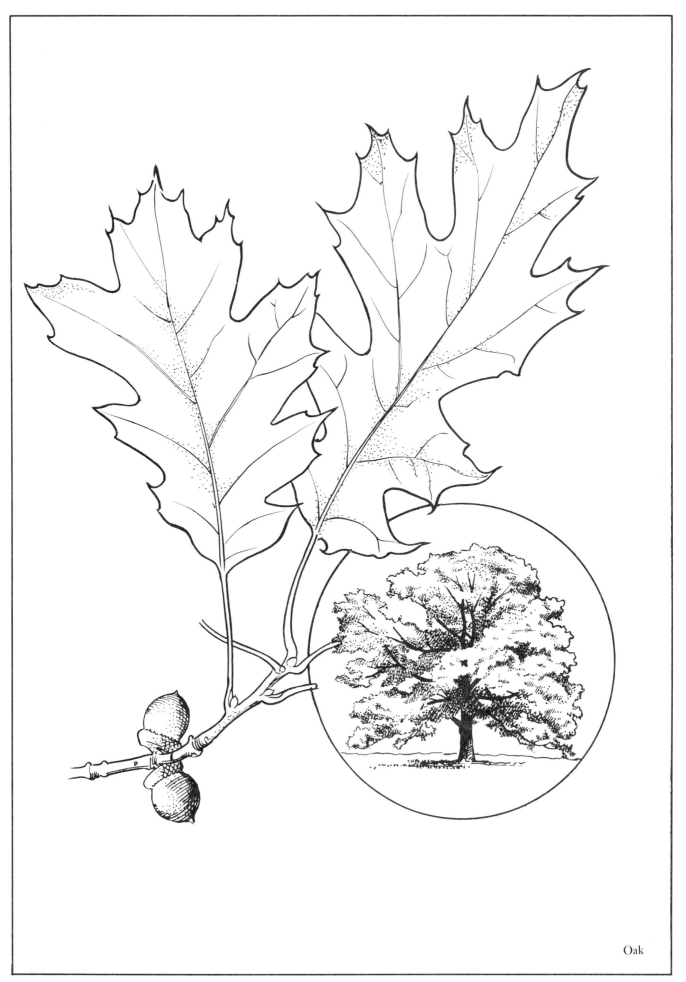

OAK

Aliases: Latin name *Quercus robur*. *Quercus* was the original common name used by the Romans; *robur*—hardness or firmness—like our word robust. Also called Jove's Tree, as it was sacred to Jove.

Companies making the essence: Bach, FES, Healing Herbs, Pegasus.

Essence qualities: Oak is a great balm to those whose lives have been a hard battle. Usually these are hardy, courageous folks, who continue to strive without complaint, but at some point they become tired and disheartened from the struggle.

Lore: A tree highly sacred to the Romans, Norse, Druids, and Celts, variously dedicated to Zeus, Jupiter, Jove, and Thor. The Celts considered it the king of trees and would build altars under it and listen to its rustling leaves for messages. It was also burned for purification. Acorns were a symbol of fertility and the continuity of life. Birthday flower for January 24, oak symbolizes courage, faith, longevity.

What the plant is like: A large hardwood tree growing to 100′ (30 m) or more tall. It has flowers, catkins, and acorns. The tree retains its leaves long after other trees have lost theirs, sometimes all winter.

Uses: The timber is valuable for furniture, buildings, and ships. The bark was used for tanning leather and fur and also as a cure for lung complaints. Oak galls, lumps secreted onto the leaf by insects, were used for ink. The acorns were used for both animal and human food, especially by Nordic peoples. In southern France, pigs are fattened on acorns, and then the fat is used to create delicate flower perfumes.

Reflections: From the reverence in which our ancestors held this tree we can see that Oak is a major restorative essence. It is especially useful in hard times and for dealing with stress.

Affirmations: I RELEASE THE EXPERIENCE OF STRUGGLE FROM MY LIFE.

I REMAIN SOLID AND STRONG IN THE FACE OF ADVERSITY.

I HAVE ALL THE STRENGTH I NEED FOR MY TASKS.

Astrological correlations: I've always thought of it as a remedy for Saturnian types, but the lore says it was sacred to the god Jupiter. (Could it take Saturnians and turn them into Jupiterians?)

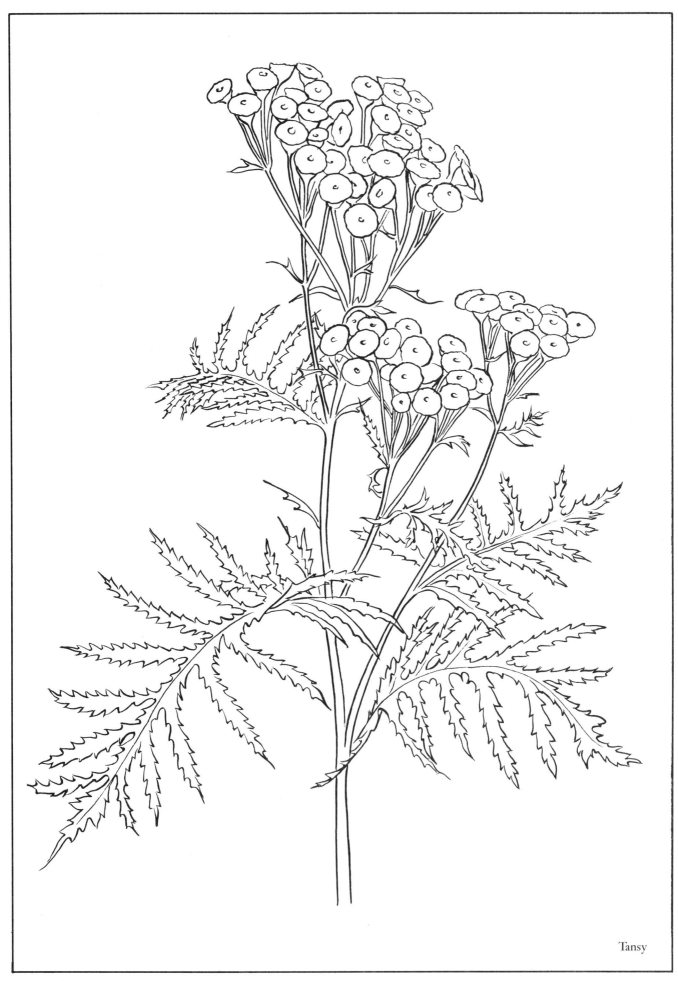

Tansy

TANSY

Aliases: Latin name *Tanacetum vulgare*. *Tanacetum* is from the medieval name for the herb, thought to be a corruption of the Greek word for immortality. *Vulgare* means common or garden variety. A popular name was buttons.

Companies making the essence: FES, Pegasus.

Essence qualities: FES says that it cuts through lethargy and sluggishness, so that one takes decisive action to meet goals.

Lore: Mentioned as early as 5000 B.C., it was considered an herb of immortality and was one of the herbs used in embalming and in purging the temple for a funeral. (The tannic acid it contained apparently did act against decay.) It was associated with Easter and was added to the batter for small cakes called tansies eaten during Lent as a symbol of everlasting life. It was also considered sacred to Mary and other goddesses and was used in women's rites. In the language of flowers, it meant, "I declare war against you." Birthday flower for February 23.

What the plant is like: Tansy is a perennial herb, growing to 3′ (1 m). In medieval Europe, it was widely cultivated for its medicinal properties; in the United States, it escaped from early settlers' gardens and became a widespread weed, growing in dry soils along roadsides. It blooms from mid- to late summer, in umbrella-like sprays of bright yellow, flat-topped blossoms. It has a medicinal odor, something like camphor.

Uses: Herbally, it was drunk as a tea and applied externally as a liniment for skin trouble, arthritis, gout, sprains, and swellings. It was used to bring a fever down and to expel worms from the body. It was kept near food as its odor repelled ants and flies. Country folk made wine from it. Because of its preservative powers, it was rubbed on meat to keep it from spoiling. The essential oil is powerful and can be poisonous in excess.

Reflections: Tansy's connections with immortality make me wonder if it would be helpful to those with terminal illnesses, giving them the emotional strength to go forward and complete the things they need to do. It should be useful also for depressed people.

Affirmations: I HAVE ALL THE STRENGTH I NEED.

TODAY I MAKE AN EFFORT.

I FINISH MY TASKS WITH EASE.

Astrological correlations: Useful for people whose Mars, the planet of energy, has difficult aspects, such as those to Saturn or Neptune. It could also help sustain those going through difficult transits to natal Mars.

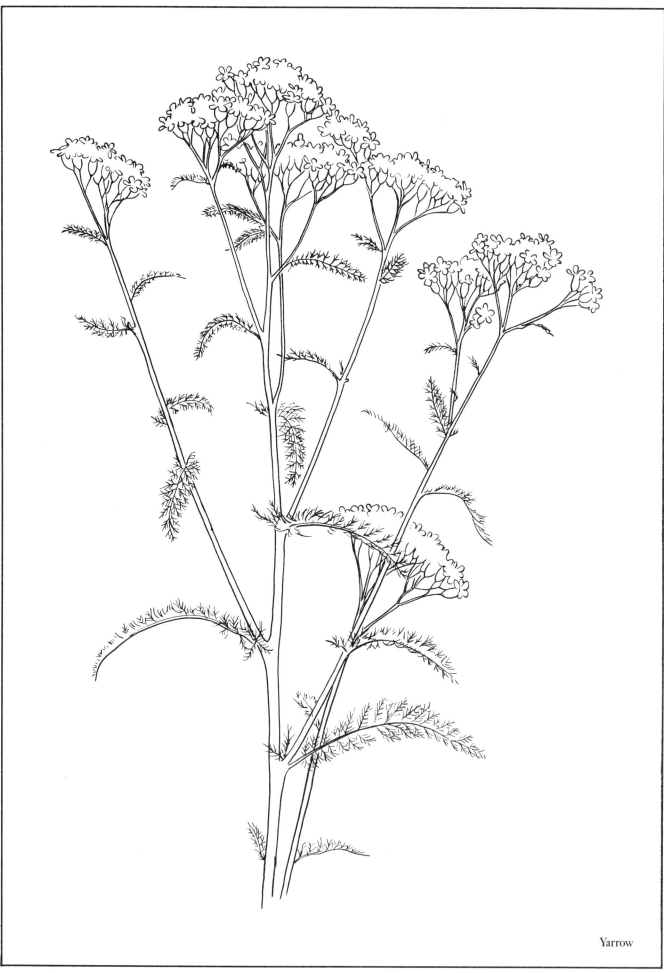

Yarrow

YARROW

Aliases: Latin name *Achillea millefolium*. *Millefolium*, as it has "thousands" of petals; *Achillea* because Achilles supposedly used this herb to stop the bleeding of his soldiers' wounds during wars. Common names abound for this once universally regarded herb, many after its healing uses: clary herb, devil's nettle, milfoil, nosebleed, sanguinary, stanch weed, and woundwort, to name just a few.

Companies making the essence: Alaskan Flower Essence Project, FES, Harebell, Pegasus, Perelandra.

Essence qualities: This essence is extremely useful for psychic shielding.

Lore: Yarrow sticks were used by the Chinese for divination, and the most prized sticks were those that grew on Confucius' grave. It was also worn for protection. Dishes or wreaths of yarrow were used by witches to keep negative energy away. Consumed as a tea, yarrow was believed to improve psychic powers. It was also supposed to attract love when carried. It was used in wedding decorations to ensure that the marriage would last at least seven years, so was also called "seven years' love." Birthday flower for January 16, it symbolized heartache and care.

What the plant is like: Tall stalks, anywhere from 2′ to 5′ (.6 to 1.5 m), on which rest sprays of tiny white or yellow flowers. It flowers late, even at the end of August.

Uses: As a poultice, the herb stopped wounds from bleeding and kept infection and swelling down. Used in beers, it gave an intoxicating quality as well as bitterness. The oil was an old remedy against baldness. A decoction in wine helped people who couldn't keep their food down. Yarrow was widely used by Native American tribes for a wide variety of illnesses. It was considered helpful against cramps and as a blood purifier.

Reflections: The centuries-long association of this plant with protection against negativity is revealed in descriptions of the essence by its makers and borne out in my experience as well. I often include it for the psychic component of codependency.

Affirmations: I MAKE CLEAR BOUNDARIES BETWEEN
MYSELF AND OTHERS.
I AM ALWAYS SAFE AND PROTECTED.

Astrological correlations: Neptune has to do with psychic abilities. Thus the person with Neptune aspects to the Ascendant, Mercury, or the Moon often has a difficult time with psychic shielding and may benefit from Yarrow.

An End—And a Beginning

Remedies alone can't magically transform our life and take all our troubles away, but what a fine addition they make! So, although this book is at an end, I hope it will be only the beginning of your happy exploration of this gentle, fascinating tool.

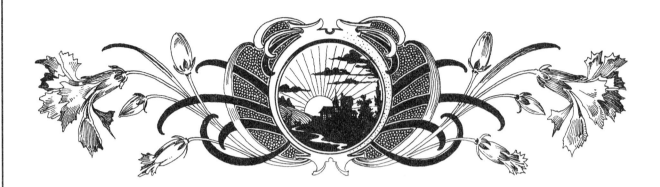

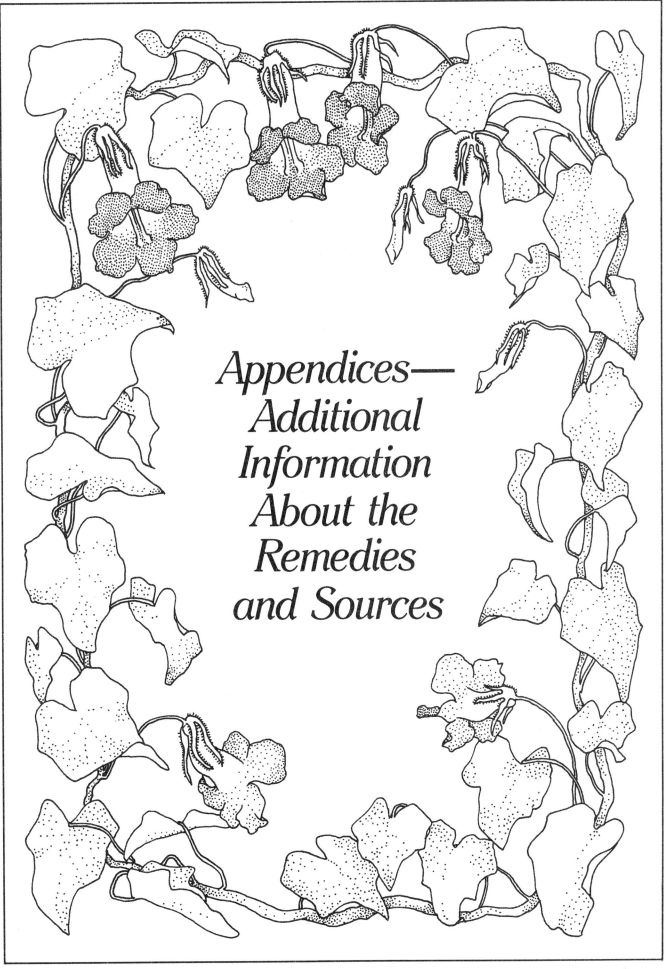

*Appendices—
Additional
Information
About the
Remedies
and Sources*

Appendix A. Flower Remedy Sources

The following are the flower essence sources currently known to me. Descriptions of a number of them can be found in chapter 2 and Appendix B. Most sources will send catalogues on request, although it would be well to enclose a dollar or two to avoid delays, as there is sometimes a charge. Many offer essence consultations by mail.

Alaskan Flower Essence Project
P.O. Box 1369
Homer, AK 99603-1369

Australian Bush Flower Essences
8A Oaks Avenue
Dee Why, NSW 2099
Australia

Ellon/Bach U.S.A., Inc.
644 Merrick Road
Lynbrook, NY 11563

Bach Flower Remedies, Ltd.
The Bach Centre
Mt. Vernon, Sotwell
Wallingford, Oxon OX1O OPZ
England

The Bailey Essences
7/8 Nelson Road
Ilkley, West Yorkshire
LS29 8HN England

Desert Alchemy
Box 44189
Tucson, AZ 85733

Deva Natural Labs Co.
Box 229
Encinitas, CA 92024

Earthfriends
Box 8468
Atlanta, GA 30306

Flower Essence Services
Box 1769
Nevada City, CA 95959

Harebell Remedies
6 Riverbank Wynd
Gatehouse of Fleet
Castle Douglas DG7 2EA
Scotland

Healing Herbs
P.O. Box 65
Hereford HR2 OUW
England

Laboratoires Deva
BP3
38880 Autrans
France

Living Essences
Box 355
Scarborough, Western Australia
Australia 6019

Master's Flower Essences
14618 Tyler Foote Road
Nevada City, CA 95959

Pacific Essences
Box 8317
Victoria, B.C.
V8W 3R9 Canada

Pegasus Products
Box 228
Boulder, CO 80306

Perelandra, Ltd.
Box 3603
Warrenton, VA 22186

Petite Fleur Essences, Inc.
8524 Whispering Creek Trail
Fort Worth, TX 76134

Santa Fe Flower Connection
Box 25
Torreon, NM 87061

Vita Florum, Ltd.
Coombe Castle, Elworthy
Taunton, Somerset TA4 3PX
England

Vita Florum
Box 876
Banff, Alberta
Canada

Appendix B.
Companies Not Already Described

Because of space limitations, the following flower essence companies were not described in chapter 2, but are reputable sources of remedies. Apparently, there are more than 40 such companies, but I am not familiar with them all. In the descriptions I indicate the degree to which I have had contact with the companies, their products, and their founders. The designation "not well known to me" does not imply anything other than that—nor does omission from this list mean anything more than that I do not yet know the company. For addresses, consult Appendix A.

The Bailey Essences: Dr. Arthur Bailey, a well-respected British dowser, became interested in testing through dowsing whether flowers other than those in the Bach kit had healing properties. Over of period of 20 years, he developed a set of 36 remedies to help people let go of unbalanced attitudes. They include flowers such as Witch Hazel, for those who try to live up to the expectations of others, and Sumac, for those who ignore their own potentials, even though they are aware of them at a deeper level. (Not well known to me.)

Desert Alchemy: These remedies are made from cacti and other desert plants, which must have a potent vital force in order to survive the harsh conditions of desert life. More than 70 well-described individual essences are available, as well as dozens of combinations. The names alone tell the story for many of these: A Way to the Elf, Celebration of Abundance, Embracing Humanness, Making and Honoring Boundaries, and Crisis-Desert Emergency Formula. Interesting and helpful astrological combinations are available for the outer planets and for the house axes.

Cofounder Cynthia Kemp, who is an astrologer, healer, and author of *Flower Essences: Bridges to the Soul*, offers workshops around the United States as well as consultations. (Well known to me.)

Earthfriends: These unique products are high-quality oils which combine flower essences and aromatherapy. They can be placed on body parts or the chakras, and the body then absorbs the essence. Added to massage oils, they can be a special way for body workers to use the essences with their clients. Several different sets are available, or oils can be ordered individually. As the founder, John Stowe, is also an astrologer, there is a set of planetary oils, for everything from the Sun to Pluto, including Chiron, and one for smooth transits. Also very powerful are the chakra balancing oils.

For those who wish to understand the chakras better as well as how to heal them, Mr. Stowe has written a clear guide, *Handbook of the Chakra Balancing Oils*. Finally, their flower meditation oils are aimed at such desirable goals as abundance, healing the child within, and dream work. Since no alcohol at all is used and the oils are not ingested, the person in recovery or those with food allergies might find them most comfortable to use. (Well known to me.)

Harebell Remedies: These delightfully old-fashioned wildflowers from the Scottish heaths make some very fine essences. Ellie Web, the founder, has a gentle, creative approach, as seen in her affirmations and the hand-drawn flower pictures on the labels. The more than 65 remedies include some duplicates of U.S. kits, and it is interesting to see the differences and similarities in the descriptions, as they evolved quite separately. Well known to me. In my work, I wouldn't be without Rhubarb, for boundaries, Heatsease for healing heartache, and Cymbidium, for embracing the tiger within.

Healing Herbs: Julian and Martine Barnard, the founders, wrote the excellent book *The Healing Herbs of Dr. Edward Bach*. The kit includes essences of the 38 flowers which were discovered and researched by Dr. Bach. Energetically sensitive people will find this set potent. FES distributes Healing Herbs in the United States. (Well known to me.)

Master's Flower Essences: Yogananda taught that foods possess actual psychological qualities that can heal us. Lila Devi Case, a longtime student of his works, developed 20 essences based on fruits and vegetables. They include such qualities as Orange, to dispel melancholia, Pear for peacefulness, and Raspberry for kindheartedness and forgiveness. Her excellent leaflet "Master's Flower Essences for Children" suggests that the essences (both of foods children especially love or crave and those they hate) can help these little ones let go of problem behaviors and develop positive new habits.

Pacific Essences: This Canadian company offers three kits totaling 36 flower essences and a set of gem elixirs. They also have an unusual kit based on sea creatures like Barnacle for trust and attunement to the physical, Sand Dollar to disrupt the mirage, and Starfish for grief and for willingly letting go of the old. (Not to worry—no sea creatures are destroyed in making the essences!) The founder, Sabina Pettitt, has also been involved with combining remedies with acupuncture and with research into the effectiveness of flower essences. (Well known to me.)

Pegasus Products: A major flower remedy company in business since the 1970s, they have upwards of a thousand offerings, including at least 70 flower remedies, more than 200 gem elixirs, and combination formulas. They have most remedies available in other kits and also serve as an American distributor for European and Australian companies. (Well known to me.)

Perelandra, Ltd.: This experienced and well-respected company has a deeply spiritual orientation. Their small but solidly researched offering includes 18 essences from common garden vegetables and flowers, and eight from roses. Their land is a nature sanctuary and research center, with nearly two tons of crystals buried in the gardens to enhance the growth of the plants and the spiritual communion with them. Educational seminars are held on the property each spring, summer, and fall. Founder Machaelle Wright has written a book, *Flower Essences*, which is a thorough, readable, and informative guide to numerous applications of the essences. An important Perelandra

remedy is Comfrey, to repair soul damage occurring in the present or a past lifetime. (Well known to me.)

Petite Fleur: A Texas-based company, founded by herbologist Judy Griffin, who has a Ph.D. in nutrition. The selection includes 84 essences, many of them from common garden flowers. Their Antique Rose Collection is based on rose bushes over 200 years old. Uses of the essences are detailed in Judy Griffin's book *Returning to the Source*. In my work with clients, I often call upon their African Violet, which releases love and nurturing from the Higher Self, Orchid, to help make peace with the past, and Japanese Magnolia, to help women resolve conflict. Their other remedies are not well known to me.

Santa Fe Flower Connection: I have no information on this company except for their brochure, written by founder Shelley Summers. They offer combinations for each chakra, for the developmental tasks and life passages of various age groups, for various emotions, and for attitudinal healing. Descriptions of each combination are included. They draw from over 230 remedies.

Vita Florum: This is an unusual combination formula made from living wild flowers, by a secret method developed by Elizabeth Bellhouse. It is "free from all violence to plants." This one all-purpose combination, intuitively derived, is said to revitalize the total being and thus to have a powerful effect on a great many medical conditions. The preparation is available in liquid, tablet, talcum, lotion, and ointment form, so that it can be directly applied to the site of the difficulty. As I do not work with medical conditions, I have no experience of this product, but Vita Florum's effects have been documented through Kirlian photography and muscle stress tests.

—— Appendix C. A Master List of Remedies ——

REMEDY	COMPANIES WHO MAKE IT	SEE CHAPTERS
African Violet	PF	3, 5, 9, Appendix
Agrimony	Bach, HH, PG	6 (profile)
Aloe Vera	DA, FES, PG	3, 4 (profile), 7, 9
Alpine Azalea	AFEP	2, 5, 8, 9
Ancestral Patterns	DA	4
Anchor Manifestation	DA	9
Arnica	DA, FES	4, 7
Aspen	Bach, DA, FES, HH	1, 3, 6
Balsam Poplar	AFEP	8
Barnacle (sea essence)	PE	Appendix
Basil	FES, PF, PG	8
Bauhinia	ABE	4
Beech	Bach, HH, PG	5, 8
Billy Goat Plum	ABE	5
Birch	FES, PG	1
Bisbee Beehive Cactus	DA	7 (profile)
Blackberry	FES, HB, MR, PG	9
Black Cohosh	DA, FES, PG	4, 7
Black-eyed Susan	FES, PG	4, 6 (profile)
Bladderwort	AFEP	4, 7, 9
Bleeding Heart	FES, PG	3, 6, 8 (profile)
Borage	FES, HB, PG	4, 6, 9
Boronia	ABE	8
Bracken	BL	5
Bright Star	DA	8
Broccoli	PR	7
Bush Gardenia	ABE	8
Bush Iris	ABE	9
Buttercup	BL, FES, PG	5 (profile), 9

ABE = Australian Bush Flower Essences
AFEP = Alaskan Flower Essence Project
BL = Bailey
DA = Desert Alchemy
FES = Flower Essence Society
HB = Harebell
HH = Healing Herbs

LE = Living Essences
MR = Master's
PE = Pacific Essences
PF = Petite Fleur
PG = Pegasus
PR = Perelandra
VF = Vitaflorum

REMEDY	COMPANIES WHO MAKE IT	SEE CHAPTERS
Calendula	FES, PG	8, 9
California Poppy	FES, PG	4, 9
California Wild Rose	FES	9
Cannabis Indica	Experimental	4
Cayenne	FES, PG	4, 8
Celebration of Abundance	DA	9
Centaury	Bach, HH, PG	7 (profile)
Chamomile	FES, PF, HB, PG	2
Chaparral	DA, FES, PG	4
Cherry Plum	Bach, HH, PG	6, 9
Chestnut Bud	Bach, HH, PG	4
Chicory	Bach, FES, HH, PG	3, 4, 5, 8
Chives	PR	8
Clematis	Bach, DA, HH, PG	6, 9
Cliff Rose	DA	9
Cognis	ABE	2, 9
Columbine	AFEP, FES, PG	5 (profile)
Comfrey	FES, HB, PG, PR	7 (profile), Appendix
Connecting With Purpose	DA	9
Corn	FES, MR, PG	9
Correa	LE	5
Crab Apple	Bach, FES, HH, PG	1, 2, 4, 5, 6, 7
Creativity Formula	DA	9
Crown of Thorns	DA, PG	8
Cymbidium	HB	5, 8, 9, Appendix
Cytisis	HB	9
Dagger Hakea	ABE	6
Dandelion	AFEP, DA, FES, HB, PG	4, 9
Deer Brush	DA, FES	6
Dill	FES, HB, PF, PG, PR	9
Dogwood	DA, FES, PG	8 (profile)

ABE = Australian Bush Flower Essences
AFEP = Alaskan Flower Essence Project
BL = Bailey
DA = Desert Alchemy
FES = Flower Essence Society
HB = Harebell
HH = Healing Herbs

LE = Living Essences
MR = Master's
PE = Pacific Essences
PF = Petite Fleur
PG = Pegasus
PR = Perelandra
VF = Vitaflorum

REMEDY	COMPANIES WHO MAKE IT	SEE CHAPTERS
Dryandra	LE	5
Elm	Bach, HH, PG	9
Embracing Humanness	DA	Appendix
Emergency Essence	ABE	2, 3
Emergency Formula	DA	2, 6, Appendix
Emotional Awareness Formula	DA	6
Fig	FES, MR, PG	1, 8, 9
Fireweed	AFEP, PG, PE	3, 4, 6
Flag Flower	LE	6
Forget-Me-Not	FES, HB, PG	1, 4, 9
Fringed Violet	ABE	7, 9
Fuchsia	FES, HB, PE, PG	4 (profile), 9
Fulfilling Your Divine Mission	DA	9
Garlic	FES	6, 9
Gentian	Bach, HH, PG	4, 5, 9
Golden Corydalis	AFEP	4, 5
Golden Eardrops	FES	5, 7
Goldenrod	FES, PG	4, 5
Gorse	Bach, HH, PG	1, 4, 9
Green Bells of Ireland	AFEP, PG	3, 9
Green Rose	LE, PG	Appendix
Grey Spider Flower	ABE	6
Harmonizing Addictive Patterns	DA	Appendix
Heartsease	HB	1, 8 (profile)
Heather	Bach, HB, HH, PG	5
Hibiscus	FES, PG	8
Holly	Bach, FES, HH, PG	1, 2, 3, 4 (profile), 6, 7
Honeysuckle	Bach, HH, PG	1, 5, 6, 8, 9
Hornbeam	Bach, HH, PG	3, 6, 9
Hound's Tongue	FES	9
Illyarrie	LE	4, 6
Impatiens	Bach, HH, PG	4, 6
Indian Paintbrush	DA, FES, PF, PG	9
Indian Pink	FES, PG	9

REMEDY	COMPANIES WHO MAKE IT	SEE CHAPTERS
Indian Pipe	PG	5
Iris	FES, PG	1, 4, 9 (profile)
Isopogon	ABE	6
Japanese Magnolia	PF	5, 8
Kapok Bush	ABE	4
Labrador Tea	AFEP	9
Lady's Mantle	HB, PG	7, 9
Larch	Bach, HH, PG	5,9
Larkspur	FES, PE, PG	4, 5
Lavender	FES, HB, PG	1, 9
Little Flannel Flower	ABE	4, 9
Lotus	FES, PG	9 (profile)
Madia	FES, PG	1, 4, 7, 9
Making and Honoring Boundaries	DA	8
Mala Mujer	DA	8
Mallow	FES, PG	8
Manzanita	FES, PG	7, 9
Mariposa Lily	DA, FES	4, 7, 8, 9
Mauve Melaleuca	LE	8
Milky Nipple Cactus	DA	4, 7
Mimulus	Bach, FES, HH, PG	4, 6
Money Plant	PG	9
Mountain Devil	ABE	6
Mountain Pride	FES, PG	9
Mountain Wormwood	AFEP	2, 6, 7, 8
Mugwort	FES, HB, PG	9
Mullein	DA, FES, PG	5 (profile), 9
Mustard	Bach, HH, PG	6
Nasturtium	BL, DA, FES, HB, PG, PR	9

ABE = Australian Bush Flower Essences
AFEP = Alaskan Flower Essence Project
BL = Bailey
DA = Desert Alchemy
FES = Flower Essence Society
HB = Harebell
HH = Healing Herbs

LE = Living Essences
MR = Master's
PE = Pacific Essences
PF = Petite Fleur
PG = Pegasus
PR = Perelandra
VF = Vitaflorum

REMEDY	COMPANIES WHO MAKE IT	SEE CHAPTERS
Northern Lights	AFEP	9
Oak	Bach, FES, HH, PG	1, 3, 4, 5, 7, 9 (profile)
Ocotillo	DA	6
Okra	FES, PG, PR	4, 9
Olive	Bach, DA, FES, HH, PG	1, 3, 6, 9
Orange	MR	Appendix
Orchid	PF	7
Oregon Grape	DA, FES, PG	4, 8
Passionflower	DA, PG	2
Pear	DA, MR	Appendix
Penstemon	FES, PG	9
Peony	FES, PE, PG	1, 8 (profile), Appendix
Philotheca	ABE	5
Pine	Bach, FES, HH, PG	1, 2, 3, 6 (profile), 8, 9
Pink Fairies	LE	6
Poison Hemlock	PE	4, 8
Poison Oak	FES	8
Polar Ice	AFEP	9
Polyanthus	PE	9
Pomegranate	DA, FES, PG	1, 8
Portage Glacier	AFEP	9
Quaking Grass	FES, PG	4
Quince	DA, FES, PG	1, 8
Raspberry	MR	Appendix
Red Chestnut	Bach, HH, PG	1, 3, 7, 8
Red Clover	BL, FES, HB, PG	6, 8
Red Helmet	ABE	7
Red Lily	ABE	9
Releasing Judgment and Denial	DA	7
Remembering and Releasing	DA	4
Rescue Remedy	Bach	3, 4, 6, 8
Rhubarb	AFEP, FES, HB, PG	8 (profile), Appendix
River Beauty	AFEP	7, 8
Rock Rose	Bach, HH, PG	6
Rosemary	DA, FES, PG	1, 7
Rose Quartz (gem elixir)	PE, PG	8

REMEDY	COMPANIES WHO MAKE IT	SEE CHAPTERS
Sagebrush	DA, FES, PG	1, 4, 5 (profile), 8
Saguaro	DA, FES, PG	5, 7, (profile), 9
St.-John's-Wort	DA, FES, HB, PG	9
Sand Dollar	PE	4, 9, Appendix
Scarlet Monkeyflower	FES	4, 6, 9
Scleranthus	Bach, HH, PG	9
Scotch Broom	FES, PG	9
Self-Heal	FES, PG	3, 4, (profile), 5
Sexual Harmony	DA	8
Shasta Daisy	FES, PG	9
Shooting Star	AFEP, FES, PG	1, 4 (profile), 9
Silver Princess	ABE	9
Sitka Burnet	AFEP	7
Snapdragon	HB	6
Soapberry	AFEP	4
Solstice Sun	AFEP	9
Southern Cross	ABE	7
Sphagnum Moss	AFEP	8
Squash	FES, PG	4, 8
Starfish (sea essence)	PE	Appendix
Star of Bethlehem	Bach, DA, HH, PG	4, 7 (profile)
Star Thistle	DA, FES	5, 9
Star Tulip	FES	9
Sticky Geranium	AFEP	4
Sticky Monkeyflower	FES	8
Strawberry Cactus	DA	9
Straw Flower Everlasting	LE	8
Sturt Desert Pea	ABE	6 (profile), 7, 8
Sumac	BL	Appendix
Sunflower	AFEP, FES, HB, PG	1, 5 (profile), 9
Sunshine Wattle	ABE	7, 9

ABE = Australian Bush Flower Essences
AFEP = Alaskan Flower Essence Project
BL = Bailey
DA = Desert Alchemy
FES = Flower Essence Society
HB = Harebell
HH = Healing Herbs

LE = Living Essences
MR = Master's
PE = Pacific Essences
PF = Petite Fleur
PG = Pegasus
PR = Perelandra
VF = Vitaflorum

REMEDY	COMPANIES WHO MAKE IT	SEE CHAPTERS
Sweet Chestnut	Bach, HH, PG	6, 8
Tall Yellow Top	ABE	4
Tansy	FES, Pegasus	9 (profile)
Tiger Lily	FES, PG	8
Transitions Formula	DA	9
Trillium	DA, FES	4, 5
Trumpet Vine	FES, PG	4, 9
Universe Handles the Details, The	DA	9
Unsealing the Akashic Records	DA	4
Unwind—Integrating Being and Doing	DA	9
Vervain	Bach, FES, HH, PG	7
Vine	Bach, HH, PG	1, 4, 7, 8
Violet	FES	4, 7
Vita Florum	VF	2, Appendix
Wallflower	FES, PG	5
Walnut	Bach, FES, HH, PG	4, 9
Watarah	ABE	6
Way to the Elf, A	DA	9
Wedding Bush	ABE	8
White Chestnut	Bach, HH, PG	2
White Narcissus	HB	9
Whitethorn	DA	9
Wild Grape	DA	8
Wild Oat	Bach, DA, HH	9
Wild Rose	Bach, HH, PG	9
Willow	Bach, FES, HH, PG	1, 2, 3, 6 (profile), 7, 9
Wisteria	ABE	8
Witch Hazel	BL	Appendix
Yarrow	AFEP, DA, FES, HB, PG, PR	1, 8, 9 (profile)
Yellow Cone Flower	LE	5
Yellow Dryas	AFEP	5
Yerba Santa	DA, FES, PG	4, 6
Zinnia	FES, PG	9

Appendix D.

Remedies for Recovery—How the Flowers Help You Work the Steps

Charlotte's Story:

Although I had been sober in Alcoholics Anonymous for several years, I had never gotten around to working the program's twelve steps. My life was still unmanageable, with one crisis or drama after another. Finally, my sponsor got tough with me. She said that if I really wanted to recover and not just be a dry drunk, I had to work the steps.

Having used up all my excuses, I turned to *The Twelve Steps and Twelve Traditions*, A.A.'s guidebook, and read each of the chapters. What a tall order, as they say in the rooms! I got to thinking which of my flower remedies could support me in working each step, and, as they really did help me through the process, I wanted to share them with other people in recovery. I would also recommend that you read the book, available at almost any Twelve-Step meeting or the public library. The steps are the same in most of these programs, helping you recover from whatever your addiction or compulsion may be. The recovery IS in the steps!

STEP ONE: WE ADMITTED WE WERE POWERLESS OVER _____ — THAT OUR LIVES HAD BECOME UNMANAGEABLE. Broccoli, by Perelandra, for confronting the feeling of powerlessness. California Poppy, by FES, for those who need to get high or to escape through drugs or alcohol. Desert Alchemy offers a combination for Harmonizing Addictive Patterns. Green Rose, by Living Essences, for the addictive personality.

STEP TWO: CAME TO BELIEVE THAT A POWER GREATER THAN OURSELVES COULD RESTORE US TO SANITY. Bach's Sweet Chestnut, for the dark night of the soul, of which hitting bottom is surely an example. St.-John's-Wort, by FES, for trust in divine protection and guidance.

STEP THREE: MADE A DECISION TO TURN OUR WILL AND OUR LIVES OVER TO THE CARE OF GOD AS WE UNDERSTOOD HIM. Fig, by FES, for trust in relationships, here with a Higher Power. Saguaro, by FES, for dealing with conflict regarding authority and power and for appreciation of the wisdom of Spirit.

STEP FOUR: MADE A SEARCHING AND FEARLESS MORAL INVENTORY OF OURSELVES. Black-eyed Susan, by FES, for resistance to looking at deep emotions and the darker side of the soul. Bach's Crab Apple, to heal shame and self-disgust. Madia, by FES, to follow through.

STEP FIVE: ADMITTED TO GOD, TO OURSELVES AND TO AN-OTHER HUMAN BEING THE EXACT NATURE OF OUR WRONGS. Cymbidium, by Harebell, for fear of disapproval. Petite Fleur's Orchid, for making peace with the past. Bach's Honeysuckle, for letting go of the past.

STEP SIX: WERE ENTIRELY READY TO HAVE GOD REMOVE ALL THESE DEFECTS OF CHARACTER. Bach's Holly will help release the most negative of character flaws. Pacific's Poison Hemlock helps you move through transitions without getting stuck.

STEP SEVEN: HUMBLY ASKED HIM TO REMOVE OUR SHORT-COMINGS. FES's Sunflower replaces false pride with a humble self-love.

STEP EIGHT: MADE A LIST OF ALL PERSONS WE HAD HARMED AND BECAME WILLING TO MAKE AMENDS TO THEM ALL. Alaska's Mountain Wormwood, for healing unforgiven areas, both towards yourself and others. Bach's Pine helps you deal with the guilt.

STEP NINE: MADE DIRECT AMENDS TO SUCH PEOPLE WHENEVER POSSIBLE, EXCEPT WHEN TO DO SO WOULD IN-JURE THEM OR OTHERS. FES's Borage gives you courage to face hard tasks cheerfully. Their Dogwood for gentleness and grace in relationships. Their Mariposa Lily, to heal alienation and separation.

STEP TEN: CONTINUED TO TAKE PERSONAL INVENTORY AND WHEN WE WERE WRONG PROMPTLY ADMITTED IT. Bach's Chestnut Bud, for learning from your mistakes and not repeating un-wanted patterns. Their Gentian, for when you have a setback or regression.

STEP ELEVEN: SOUGHT THROUGH PRAYER AND MEDITA-TION TO IMPROVE OUR CONSCIOUS CONTACT WITH GOD AS WE UNDERSTOOD HIM, PRAYING ONLY FOR KNOWLEDGE OF HIS WILL FOR US AND THE POWER TO CARRY THAT OUT. Lotus, by FES, is the best spiritual support. Their Hound's Tongue uplifts the overmaterialistic. Corn, to balance heaven and earth.

STEP TWELVE: HAVING HAD A SPIRITUAL AWAKENING AS THE RESULT OF THESE STEPS, WE TRIED TO CARRY THIS MESSAGE TO ALCOHOLICS AND TO PRACTICE THESE PRIN-CIPLES IN ALL OUR AFFAIRS. Golden Corydalis, by Alaska, to reinte-grate the personality after a deep transformation. FES's Trillium, for working for the common good.

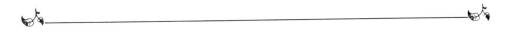

Appendix E. Bibliography

I. BOOKS ABOUT FLOWER ESSENCES

Alaskan Flower Essence Project. Flower Essence Studies. Fairbanks: The Alaskan Flower Essence Project, 1989.

Bach, Edward, M.D., and F. J. Wheeler, M.D. *The Bach Flower Remedies*. New Canaan, CT: Keats Publishing, Inc., 1979.

———. *The Twelve Healers and Other Remedies*. Saffron Walden, England: The C. W. Daniel Co. Ltd., 1976.

Barnao, Va'sudeva. *Healing with Australian Flowers*. Perth, Western Australia: Living Essences, 1988. (Box 355, Scarborough, Perth, Western Australia 6019)

Barnard, Julian and Martine. *The Healing Herbs of Edward Bach: an Illustrated Guide to the Flower Remedies*. Hereford, England: The Bach Educational Programme, 1988.

Bellhouse, Elizabeth. *Measureless Healing*. Taunton, Somerset, England: The Elizabeth Bellhouse Foundation, 1985. (Re: Vita Florum.)

Chancellor, Dr. Philip M. *Handbook of the Bach Flower Remedies*. Saffron Walden, England: The C. W. Daniel Co. Ltd., 1976.

Damian, Peter. *The Twelve Healers of the Zodiac*. York Beach, ME: Samuel Weiser, Inc., 1986.

Flower Essence Society. *The Flower Essence Repertory*. Nevada City, CA: The Flower Essence Society, rev. ed., 1992.

———. *Healing Today's Child: the Magic of Flower Essences*. Nevada City, CA: The Flower Essence Society, 1987. (monograph)

Griffin, Judy. *Returning to the Source*. Ft. Worth, TX: Petite Fleur Essence, Inc., rev. ed., 1989. (Re: their essences)

Gurudas. *Flower Essences and Vibrational Healing*. San Rafael, CA: Cassandra Press, rev. ed., 1988.

Hyne Jones, T. W. *Dictionary of the Bach Flower Remedies: Positive and Negative Aspects*. Saffron Walden, England: The C. W. Daniel Co. Ltd., 1976. (42 pp.)

Kemp, Cynthia. *Flower Essences: Bridges to the Soul*. Tucson, AZ: Desert Alchemy, 1988. (monograph)

Krishnamurti, V. *Beginner's Guide to the Bach Flower Remedies*. New Delhi, India: B. Jain Publishers Ltd., 1988.

Rotella, Alexis. *The Essence of Flowers: New Age Wisdom*. Mountain Lakes, NJ: Jade Mountain Press, 1990.

Starck, Marcia. *Earth Mother Astrology*. St. Paul, MN: Llewellyn Publications, 1989.

Vlamis, Gregory. *Flowers to the Rescue: The Healing Vision of Dr. Edward Bach*. Rochester, VT: Healing Arts Press, 1988.

Weeks, Nora. *The Medical Discoveries of Edward Bach*. New Canaan, CT: Keats Publishing, 1979.

White, Ian. *Australian Bush Flower Essences*. Sydney, Australia: Bantam Books, 1991.

Wood, Matthew. *Seven Herbs: Plants as Teachers*. Berkeley, CA: North Atlantic Books, 1987.

Wright, Machaelle Small. *Flower Essences*. Warrenton, VA: Perelandra Ltd., 1988.

II. BOOKS ON HERBALISM

Beyerl, Paul. *The Master Book of Herbalism*. Custer, WA: Phoenix Publishing Co., 1984. (Order from Phoenix, Box 10, Custer, WA 98240)

Culpeper, Nicholas. *Culpeper's Herbal Remedies*. North Hollywood, CA: Wilshire Book Company, 1971.

Cunningham, Scott. *Cunningham's Encyclopedia of Magical Herbs*. St. Paul, MN: Llewellyn Publications, 1989.

Ericksen-Brown, Charlotte. *Medicinal and Other Uses of North American Plants*. New York: Dover Publications, Inc., 1989.

Kresanek, Dr. Jaroslav. *Healing Plants*. New York: Dorset Press, 1989.

Leung, Albert Y. *Chinese Herbal Remedies*. New York: Universe Books, 1974.

Levy, Juliette de Bairacli. *Common Herbs for Natural Health*. New York: Schocken Books, 1974.

Mestel, Sherry, ed. *Earth Rites*, Volume 1: *Herbal Remedies*. New York: Earth Rites Press, 1980.

Meyer, David C., ed. *The Herbalist Almanac: 50-Year Anthology*. Glenwood, IL: Meyerbooks, 1988.

Meyer, Joseph E. *The Herbalist*. Glenwood, IL: Meyerbooks, rev. ed., 1986.

Mills, Simon. *The Dictionary of Modern Herbalism.* Rochester, VT: Healing Arts Press, 1988.

Miluck, Melva M., and Carol Hovin. *Twelve Herbs of Light.* Bozeman, MT: Clarestar, 1986.

Muir, Ada. *The Healing Herbs of the Zodiac.* St. Paul, MN: Llewellyn Publications, 1988.

Tenney, Louise. *Today's Herbal Health.* Provo, UT: Woodland Books, 1983.

III. BOOKS ON GARDENING, FLOWERS, AND PLANTS

Art, Henry W. *A Garden of Wildflowers.* Pownal, VT: Storey Communications, Inc., 1986.

Coombes, Allen J. *Dictionary of Plant Names.* Portland, OR: Timber Press, 1985.

Houk, Rose. *Eastern Wildflowers.* San Francisco: Chronicle Books, 1989.

Macoboy, Stirling. *What Flower Is That?* New York: Portland House, rev. ed., 1988.

Murray, Liz and Colin. *The Celtic Tree Oracle.* New York: St. Martin's Press, 1988.

Okun, Sheila. *A Book of Cut Flowers.* New York: Michael Friedman Publishing Group, 1988.

Peterson, Lee Allen. *Peterson Field Guides #23: Edible Wild Plants.* Boston: Houghton Mifflin Company, 1977.

Peterson, Roger Tory, and Margaret McKenny. *Peterson Field Guides #17: Wildflowers, Northeastern/ North Central North America.* Boston: Houghton Mifflin Company, 1968.

Riotte, Louise. *Astrological Gardening.* Pownal, VT: Storey Communications, 1988.

Spencer, Edwin Rollin. *All About Weeds.* New York: Dover Publications, Inc., 1974.

Stokes, Donald and Lillian. *A Guide to Enjoying Wildflowers.* Boston: Little, Brown and Company, 1985.

IV. INFORMATION ON FLOWER HISTORY AND SYMBOLISM

Addison, Josephine. *The Illustrated Plant Lore.* Manchester, NH: Salem House, 1986.

Beyerl, Paul. *The Master Book of Herbalism.* Custer, WA: Phoenix Publishing Co., 1984.

Conway, D. J. *Celtic Magic.* St. Paul, MN: Llewellyn Publications, 1990.

Cunningham, Scott. *Cunningham's Encyclopedia of Magical Herbs.* St. Paul, MN: Llewellyn Publications, 1989.

Ewart, Neil. *The Lore of Flowers.* Dorset, England: Blandford Press, 1982. (U.S. Distributor: Sterling Publishing Co., Inc., 387 Park Ave So., New York, NY 10016.)

Greenaway, Kate, and Jean Marsh. *The Illuminated Language of Flowers.* New York: Holt, Rinehart and Winston, 1978.

Heinerman, John, Ph.D. *Spiritual Wisdom of the Native Americans.* San Rafael, CA: Cassandra Press, 1989.

Jobes, Gertrude. *Dictionary of Mythology, Folklore, and Symbols.* New York: Scarecrow Press, 1962.

Lehner, Ernst and Johanna. *Folklore and Symbolism of Flowers, Plants, and Trees.* New York: Tudor Publishing, 1960.

Meyer, Clarence. *The Herbalist Almanac: A 50-Year Anthology.* Glenwood, IL: Meyerbooks, 1977. (Order from Box 427, Glenwood, IL 60425.)

Mother, The. *Flowers and Their Messages.* Auroville, India: Sri Aurobindo Ashram Publications, enlarged ed., 1984.

Pickles, Sheila, ed. *The Language of Flowers.* New York: Harmony House, 1990.

Tompkins, Peter, and Christopher Bird. *The Secret Life of Plants.* New York: Harper and Row, 1973.

Walker, Winifred. *All the Plants of the Bible.* Garden City, NY: Doubleday & Company, 1979.

Appendix F.
Format for Profiles of the 30 Key Remedies

Aliases: Other names the plant is known by. The botanical, or Latin, name and its meaning is given first, to identify the exact species and variety of plant used in making the essence. The botanical name also frequently reflects the legends or history surrounding the plant. Next come the various common names of the plant. Many of these names reflect the plant's lore or healing uses.

Companies making the essence: listed in alphabetical order.

Essence qualities: Here, the description is usually the one that appears in the catalog or literature of the company whose product I use. Again, this is not to recommend that company over the others, only to give credit to the company in question for their understanding of the remedy.

Lore: The history, legends, symbolism, mythology, and popular beliefs about a plant. Often these have interesting correlations with the essence qualities.

What the plant is like: A brief description of the plant and flower, along with any unusual growing habits or properties. This type of information can be part of the signature of the plant.

Uses: The agricultural, culinary, medicinal, or decorative uses the plant has been put to, either currently or historically. This information has been culled from a variety of books that are listed in the bibliography. Although herbal uses are given, the methods are not described, nor should you use them without consulting with a qualified health care practitioner. Herbs can be toxic if used incorrectly and in the wrong amount.

Reflections: Ideas and associations suggested by the information given above, as well as personal experiences in the uses of the remedy.

Affirmations: Suggested affirmations to use while taking the remedy, which you would want to personalize for the situation.

Astrological correlations: Briefly, for the astrological student or professional, how to use and synchronize the remedies with an astrological chart, using natal or transiting placements.

Appendix G. Notes

Chapter 1

1. Ewart, Neil. *The Lore of Flowers*. Dorset, England: Blandford Press, 1982, p. 153.

2. Jobes, Gertrude. *Dictionary of Mythology, Folklore, and Symbols*. New York: Scarecrow Press, 1962, p. 75.

3. Jobes, op cit, pp. 1724–5.

4. Pachter, Henry M. *Magic Into Science: The Story of Paracelsus*. New York: Henry Schuman Co., 1951, p. 80.

5. Tompkins, Peter, and Christopher Bird. *The Secret Life of Plants*. New York: Harper and Row, 1973, p. 136.

6. Kraft, Ken and Pat. *Luther Burbank: The Wizard and the Man*. New York: Meredith Press, 1967, p. 124–132.

7. These experiments were reported in Shirley Ross, *Plant Consciousness and Plant Care*, New York: Quadrangle/New York Times Book Company, 1973, pp. 89–97, as well as in *The Secret Life of Plants*.

8. Addison, Josephine. *The Illustrated Plant Lore*. Manchester, N.H.: Salem House, 1986.

9. Pickles, Sheila, ed. *The Language of Flowers*. New York: Harmony House, 1990.

Chapter 2

1. As described in Simonton, Carl, *Getting Well Again*, New York: Bantam, 1982.

2. Philip M. Chancellor. *Handbook of the Bach Flower Remedies*. Saffron Walden, England: The C. W. Daniel Co. Ltd., 1976.

3. Vlamis, Gregory. *Flowers to the Rescue: The Healing Vision of Dr. Edward Bach*. Rochester, VT: Healing Arts Press, 1988.

4. The photographs originally appeared in a book that is no longer in print: Krippner, Stanley, and David Rubin. *The Kirlian Aura*. Anchor Books, New York, 1974. The book currently in print that has the best displays of Kirlian photography is *Kirlian Photography: Research and Prospects* by Luigi Gennaro, Fulvio Guzzon, and Pierluigi Marsigli, published by East-West Publications, London, 1980.

5. Vol. 1:1 (1980), pp. 11–14. Order from the Flower Essence Society, Box 459, Nevada City, CA 95959.

6. Gillemo, Ken. *Cause, Effect and Treatment*. English translation published by The Elizabeth Bellhouse Foundation, Taunton, Somerset, England, 1988, pp. 16–19.

7. Weeks, Norah. *Medical Discoveries of Edward Bach*. New Canaan, CT: Keats Publishing, 1979.

8. Wood, Matthew. *Seven Herbs: Plants as Teachers*. Berkeley, CA: North Atlantic Books, 1987.

Chapter 4

1. Flower Essence Society. *The Flower Essence Repertory*. Nevada City, CA: The Flower Essence Society, 1987, pp. 55 and 59.

2. Flower Essence Society, ibid, pp. 53 and 59.

3. Woolger, Roger. *Other Lives, Other Selves*. New York: Bantam, 1988.

4. As discussed in his article, "Flower Essences and Devic Attunement," in the *Alaskan Flower Essence Project Newsletter*, Spring 1990, p. 1.

5. Cunningham, Donna. *Moon Signs*. New York: Ballantine Books, p. 19.

Chapter 5

1. In particular, Sondra Ray's two books published by Celestial Arts are excellent: *The Only Diet There Is* (1981) and *I Deserve Love* (1987).

Chapter 6

1. Vlamis, Gregory. *Flowers to the Rescue: The Healing Vision of Dr. Edward Bach*. Rochester, VT: Healing Arts Press, 1988.

2. Alaskan Flower Essence Project. *Flower Essence Studies*. Fairbanks, AK: The Alaskan Flower Essence Project, 1989, p. 9.

3. White, Ian. *Australian Bush Flower Essences*. Sydney, Australia: Bantam Books, 1991, pp. 144–7.

Chapter 7

1. A much longer explanation of the following material is published in my chapter on ACAs and Codependency in the Joan McEvers anthology, *Astrological Counseling*. St. Paul, MN: Llewellyn, 1990.

2. Cermak, Timmen L., M.D. *A Primer for Adult Children of Alcoholics*, second ed. Deerfield Beach, FL: Health Publications, Inc., 1989, pp. 34–37.

3. These characteristics come from the incest survivors' checklist in E. Sue Blume's *Secret Survivors*. New York: John Wiley & Sons, Inc., 1990, pp. xviii–xix.

4. Flower Essence Society. *The Flower Essence Repertory*. Nevada City, CA: The Flower Essence Society, 1987, p. 72.

5. Wood, Matthew. *Seven Herbs: Plants as Teachers*. Berkeley, CA: North Atlantic Books, 1987.

Chapter 8

1. Cermak, Timmen L., M.D. *A Primer for Adult Children of Alcoholics*, second ed. Deerfield Beach, FL: Health Publications Inc., 1989, pp. 19–23.

Chapter 9

1. Flower Essence Society. *The Flower Essence Repertory*. Nevada City, CA: The Flower Essence Society, 1987, p. 59.

2. White, Ian. *Australian Bush Flower Essences*. Sydney, Australia: Bantam Books, 1991.

3. Gage Allee, John. *Webster's Dictionary*, 1988 ed. Baltimore: Ottenheimer Publishers, Inc., p. 91.

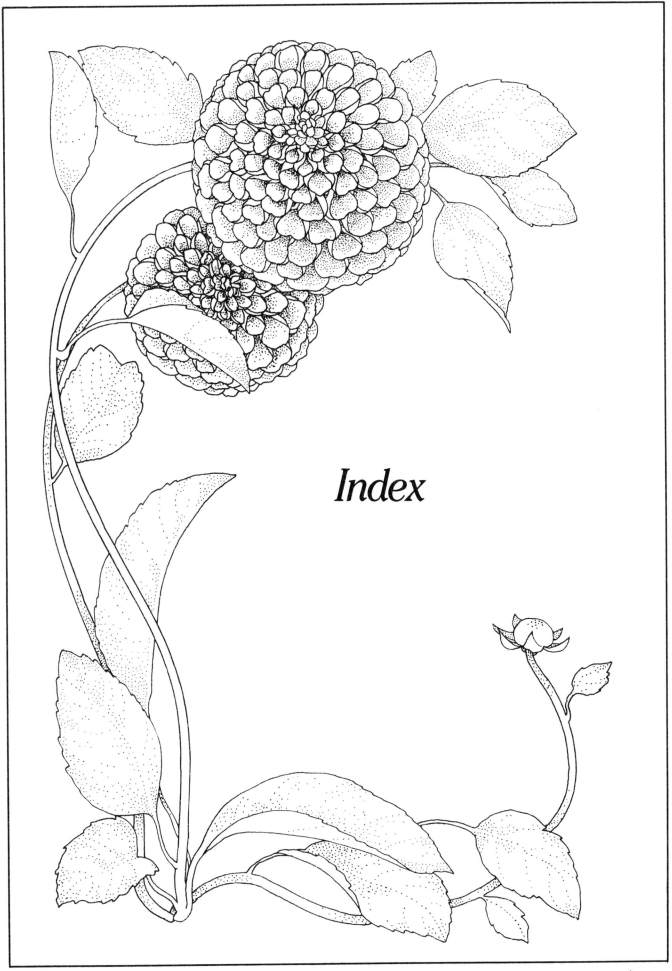

Index

INDEX

Sunflower, 12, 15, 65, 68, 69, 78–79, 130, 153, 174, 177
   in combination, 66
   related to, 93
   worship, 12, 79
Sunshine Wattle, 43, 109, 147, 151, 174
Support from eternal part of being, 144
   groups, 35, 44
Suppression of sorrow, 89
Surgery, remedies for before and after, 84
Surrendering
   personal will, 149
   to healing process, 102
Survival, 49
Survivors, 102
Suspicion, 57, 87, 126
Sweet Chestnut, 89, 125, 175, 176
Sweet pea, 12, 14
Symbolism, 37
Symphytum officinale, 115

Talent, lacking, 151
Talking too much, 141
Tall Yellow Top, 46, 175
Tanacetum vulgare, 161
Tannic acid, 161
Tansy, 14, 145, 149, 160–161, 175
Tasks, facing difficult, 177
Taste, in good, 55
Tea, 163
   self-heal, 59
Teachers, 152
Tears, 133
Tension
   chronic, 149
   release of, 48
Terror, 85
Tests, 85
   flower remedy, 26
Tetanus, 57
Thapsus, Tunisia, 75
Therapy, remedies to help, 44–45
Thoughts, unwanted, 25, 137
Throat chakra, 150
   remedy, 87
Thyroid, 141
Tickle-my-fancy, 137
Tiger, embracing the, 167
Tiger Lily, 128, 175
Timidity, 46, 84, 87
Tompkins, Peter, 22
Touch for Health, 49, 124
Touching, fear of, 48, 103
Toxic shame, 85–86
Traits
   ACAs, 104
   codependents, 131
   incest survivors, 104–105

Trance states, 113
Tranquilizers, 88
Transition, 177
   formula, 145, 175
   people in, 145
Trauma, 49, 50, 85, 103, 106, 115, 119, 153
   physical, 48
Tree calendar, 18
Trillium, 15, 46, 69, 175, 177
True to oneself, 65, 69, 75, 77, 131
Trumpet Vine, 46, 87, 146, 147, 150, 175
Trust, 44, 46, 53, 59, 126, 128, 152, 168
   in divine, 176
Turnarounds, amazing, 89
Twelve-step groups, 103
Twelve Steps and Twelve Traditions, 86, 176

Unforgiven areas, 87, 177
Unity, 119, 153
Universe Handles the Details, The, 149, 175
Unsealing the Akashic Records, 50, 175
Unwind—Integrating Being and Doing, 150, 175
Uplifting, 177
Upset about others' upheavals, 84
Upwardly mobile people, 77
Uranus, aspects and transits, 59, 61, 73, 75, 117, 119

Valuing our own gifts, 145
Venus, aspects and transits, 73, 133, 135, 137, 139
Verbascum thapsus, 75
Vervain, 15, 37, 108, 109, 175
Vibrations, to clear, 77
Victims and victimizers, 47, 103, 104, 131
Vine, 16, 18, 44, 104, 105, 127, 128, 175
Viola tricolor, 137
Violence, victim of, 47
Violet, 13, 14–15, 19, 46, 103, 175
Virginia, state flower of, 135
Virgo, strong influence in, 95
Vision, holding to a, 145
Vita Florum, 26, 166, 168, 175
Vitality, to restore, 53, 146, 151
Vlamis, Gregory, 26, 84
Vulnerability, 141

Wallflower, 15, 65, 67, 175
Walnut, 14, 46, 145, 175
Warmth, 46
Watarah, 89, 175
Water lily, 13, 15, 19
Way to the Elf, A, 151, 175
Weakness of will, 108

Web, Ellie, 167
Wedding Bush, 126, 127, 175
Wedding decorations, 163
Weeks, Norah, 27
Weeping willow, 15, 99
Weiglas, Michael, 26, 31
Well-being, to give feeling of, 85
Whiplash, 106
White Chestnut, 25, 175
White, Ian, 97, 107, 108, 147
White Narcissus, 151, 175
Whitethorn, 18, 150, 175
Wildflowers, 168
   Scottish, 167
Wild Grape, 131, 175
Wild Oat, 144, 175
Wild Rose, 147, 175
Wild pansy, 137
Willow, 11, 13, 15, 17, 18, 24, 38, 87, 89, 98–99, 108, 175
Wisteria, 129, 175
Witches, 11, 75, 113, 163
Witches' aspirin, 99
Witch Hazel, 16, 167, 175
Women's conflicts, 168
   rites, 161
Women Who Love Too Much, 122
Wood, Matt, 32, 77, 106, 108
Woolger, Dr. Roger, 49
Workaholics, 150
Worries, 25, 84
Worthiness, 148
Woundwort, 59, 163
Wright, Machaelle, 168
Wrinkle remedy, 95
Writers, 150

Yarrow, 14, 131, 153, 162–163, 175
   sticks, 11
Yellow Cone Flower, 65–66, 69, 175
Yellow Dryas, 66, 175
Yerba Santa, 32, 83, 107, 175
Yew, 14, 18
Yogananda, Paramahansa, 21, 167

Zest, 151
Zinnia, 144, 151, 175
Zodiac signs and their flowers, 19

About the Author

Donna Cunningham brings to her flower essence practice a rich background of 25 years of counselling experience and more than a decade of study of the flower remedies. She has a Master's Degree in Social Work from Columbia University. She has worked in medical settings, in women's health, in psychiatric clinics, in the treatment of people with disabilities, and with alcoholics.

She has also been an astrologer for 22 years and has won recognition for her eight previous books—two of them about recovery from addiction and the others about astrology. She gives lectures and workshops internationally and her books have been published in many foreign languages, including Portuguese, Spanish, German, Dutch, Swedish and Norwegian. In 1986, Professional Astrologers Incorporated gave her their annual award for her lifetime contributions to the field.

Donna began using flower remedies extensively with therapy and astrological clients in 1981, often doing flower remedy consultations by mail. Observations about the remedies appear in five previous books. She was invited to speak about the correlation between flower remedies and astrology at the First and Second World Flower Essence Congresses. She was also editor and publisher of *Shooting Star*, an independent quarterly for combining flower remedies and astrology.

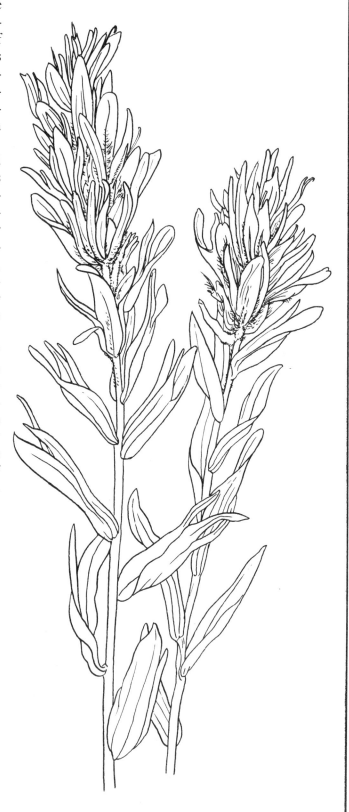

Indian Paintbrush